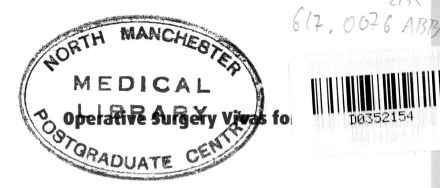

Operative Surgery Vivas for

This is a comprehensive study manual for the operative surgery
section of the MRCS examination. This unique text is set to the
level of a basic surgical examination and the material is discussed in easy to access, simple manner. The
A--Z format means topics appear, mirroring the
nature of the examination. For each operative procedure the
basic principles, applied anatomy, indications and complications are discussed alongside an overview of technique.
Frequently asked examination questions and practical tips for
giving the fullest answer for the most marks are also included.
Care has been taken to ensure compatibility with all UK syl-
labuses, and inclusion of material required for equivalent exam-
inations internationally. This manual is an excellent source of
information for use during personal study and self-testing, and
as a teaching aid.

Ali Abbassian MRCS is a Specialist Registrar in Trauma and
Orthopaedics on the North-West Thames training programme.

Sarah Krishnanandan MRCS is a Specialist Registrar in Emergency
Medicine on the South Thames training programme.

Christopher James MRCS is a Clinical Fellow in Trauma and
Orthopaedics at Guy's Hospital in London.

To Cameron and Kirsty who in their own special way have made our lives full and this book possible.

Operative Surgery Vivas for the MRCS

Ali Abbassian
Sarah Krishnanandan and
Christopher James

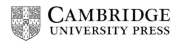

CAMBRIDGE
UNIVERSITY PRESS

CAMBRIDGE UNIVERSITY PRESS

Cambridge, New York, Melbourne, Madrid, Cape Town, Singapore, São Paulo

Cambridge University Press
The Edinburgh Building, Cambridge CB2 2RU, UK

Published in the United States of America by Cambridge University Press,
New York

www.cambridge.org
Information on this title: www.cambridge.org/9780521674416

First published 2006
Typeset by Charon Tec Ltd (A Macmillan Company), Chennai, India
www.charontec.com

Printed in the United Kingdom at the University Press, Cambridge

A catalogue record for this publication is available from the British Library

Library of Congress Cataloguing in Publication data

ISBN-13 978-0-521-67441-6 paperback
ISBN-10 0-521-67441-7 paperback

Contents

Contents

Preface

The MRCS viva examination is divided into six separate sections. These include: critical care, physiology, pathology, principles of surgery, anatomy and operative surgery. In each viva, examiners aim to include questions from at least two or three and sometimes even four or five different topics. This generally means that there are only a few minutes to discuss each topic. It is therefore important for candidates to have a broad knowledge of many aspects of surgery in general. I think in preparing for this part of the examination one should avoid focusing on intricate details of every surgical topic and instead have a simple understanding and an overview of all the basics.

Operative surgery section of the examination tests the knowledge of clinical anatomy. Be prepared to be shown bones, instruments and dissections, and to be asked to draw surface markings. You are not expected to be able to competently perform complex surgery; however, you must understand the relevant anatomy and be aware of the indications, complications and alternatives to the common surgical procedures in each surgical discipline.

In this book we have tried to include some of the more frequently asked questions. For each procedure the clinically relevant basic science is discussed and the surgical technique is outlined. Don't forget to start every answer with comments on appropriate examination, consent and positioning of the patient pre-operatively.

In my opinion anatomy is the most important part of your basic surgical training and its knowledge is pivotal to your passing the examination and later becoming a competent surgeon in your chosen speciality. Unfortunately there are no short cuts and one must learn the entire human anatomy. This is why spending some time in an anatomy demonstrating post is a good idea. I found larger textbooks easier to learn from as they tend to have more pictures and diagrams. I also strongly recommend attending reputable viva preparation courses prior to your examination.

Finally, "practice makes perfect", and that is exactly why using this book will help in improving your knowledge and increasing your confidence. Its A–Z format means that the topics appear at random and therefore provide a useful revision aid. This worked for us and I am sure it will for you. Good luck.

Ali Abbassian

1

The elective repair of an abdominal aortic aneurysm

1 What are the indications for the elective repair of an abdominal aortic aneurysm (AAA)?

According to the UK Small Aneurysm Trial the repair of asymptomatic infrarenal aneurysms between 4 and 5.5 cm in size proved to be of no survival benefit when compared to patients who just had regular ultrasound scans.

Therefore an AAA should be repaired if:

- The aneurysm is symptomatic
- The aneurysm is over 5.5 cm in size or
- The aneurysm shows a rapid rate of expansion (over 1 cm/annum)

2 What pre-operative measures should be taken?

- Investigations: These patients usually have significant co-morbidity therefore their renal, lung and cardiac function must be assessed closely with the anaesthetist. They may require lung function tests, echocardiograms, thallium scans and exercise tolerance tests.

An ultrasound scan is a useful screening tool and is also the investigation of choice for monitoring the size of an aneurysm. CT with contrast enhancement is the gold standard investigation in preparing the patient for repair since it delineates the aneurysm's anatomy and its relation to the renal arteries. Intra-arterial digital subtraction angiography (IADSA) is used in suprarenal aneurysms or in those patients with renal impairment.

- Cross-match 8 units of blood.
- Insert two venous cannulae, a catheter and an arterial line (early involvement of intensive care support).
- Peri-operative broad-spectrum antibiotics.
- Informed consent.

3 How do you perform an open repair of an AAA?

2

Position The patient is placed supine and the abdomen is prepared as for a laparotomy.

Incision Long midline laparotomy incision.

Procedure Expose the aorta (pack small bowel up to the right and dissect off the peritoneum). Define the extent of the aneurysm. Place clamps across the neck and lower end of the aneurysm. Open the sac and suture the lumbar vessels from within.

Replace the aorta between the renal arteries and the bifurcation with a Dacron prosthesis (occasionally it may be necessary to bring a "Trouser graft" down to the femoral arteries).

Cover the graft with the aneurysm sac.

Repair the peritoneum, check for distal limb pulses.

Closure This is in layers as for laparotomy (see Chapter 24, Laparotomy and abdominal incisions).

4 What are some of the complications specific to an AAA repair?

- Immediate
  - Haemorrhage
  - Distal limb embolisation (trash foot)
  - Distal limb arterial thrombosis
- Early
  - Spinal cord ischaemia
  - Acute sigmoid colon ischaemia (mesenteric)
  - Acute renal failure, myocardial infarction, cerebrovascular accident
- Late
  - False aneurysm formation
  - Graft infection
  - Aorto-duodenal fistula formation
  - Impotence

3

5 What do you know about the "endoluminal repair" of abdominal aneurysms?

This involves the introduction of an endoprosthesis into the aorta via the femoral artery under fluoroscopic guidance. The procedure requires 1.5 cm of healthy aorta proximally and 1 cm distally. Suprarenal aneurysms cannot be repaired in this way. This repair is ideal for "inflammatory" aneurysms.

The complications of endoluminal repair include: "endoleaks" (caused by back bleeding from lumbar arteries), graft migration and infection, and as with open repair, distal embolisation.

6 What is the mortality for elective AAA repairs?

The mortality rate remains at 5% (but is higher for inflammatory aneurysms).

7 What are the surface markings of the abdominal aorta?

- The abdominal aorta begins at the aortic hiatus in the diaphragm. This is at the level of the 12th thoracic vertebra or an inch above the transpyloric plane of Addison (a plane midway between the suprasternal notch and the pubic symphysis).
- It ends at the 4th lumbar vertebra, or 1.5 cm to the left of the midline at the supracristal plane (a plane joining the highest points of the iliac crests) where it bifurcates into the common iliac arteries.
- Its three unpaired branches are:
  1 T12: The coeliac axis
  2 L1: The superior mesenteric artery
  3 L3: The inferior mesenteric artery

4

8 What is the significance of the artery of Adamkiewicz?

This is a major radicular artery that supplies a great proportion of the spinal cord. It usually arises from the posterior intercostal arteries and is left sided in 80% of subjects. It can however arise from the lumbar arteries which are oversewn during an AAA repair. This may then lead to cord ischaemia and paralysis.

Adrenalectomy

1 What are the common indications for an adrenalectomy?

- Phaeochromocytoma
- Cushing's syndrome
- Conn's syndrome
- Carcinoma

2 What is the arterial supply of the adrenal glands?

The glands have a rich blood supply from three main sources:
1 The inferior phrenic artery via a number of small *superior* adrenal arteries
2 The aorta via one or more *middle adrenal* arteries
3 The renal artery via one or more *inferior adrenal* arteries

3 What is the venous drainage of the adrenal glands?

The right gland is drained via a short adrenal vein directly into the inferior vena cava (IVC). The left gland drains via a longer left adrenal vein into the left renal vein which in turn drains into the IVC. Laparoscopic dissection and clipping of the right adrenal vein is therefore more challenging than the left.

4 Peri-operative preparation of a patient prior to adrenalectomy for a phaeochromocytoma is particularly challenging. What special measures are taken?

- Pre-operative alpha (e.g. phenoxybenzamine) and beta (e.g. propanalol) blockade for at least 4 weeks
- Careful and invasive monitoring of blood pressure and volume during and after surgery
- Gentle handling of the tumour to avoid sudden release of catecholamines
- Intravenous nitrates to control hypertensive episodes during surgery
- Colloid replacement in case of hypotension

6

5 Name some of the approaches used to perform an adrenalectomy

- Transperitoneal approach: large transverse upper abdominal incision, which gives an excellent exposure. This is suitable for large or bilateral tumours.
- Thoraco-abdominal approach.
- Laparoscopic adrenalectomy.
- Posterior extra-peritoneal approach similar to the approach used for a nephrectomy.

6 List some of the complications of adrenalectomy

- General
  - Wound infection
  - Damage to surrounding organs and vessels

- Haemorrhage
- Thrombosis
- Ileus
- Incisional hernia
- Hormonal
  - Hypertensive crisis during surgery (phaeochromocytoma)
  - Hypotensive crisis following surgery (phaeochromocytoma)
  - Addisonian crisis following surgery (Cushing's)

7 When is a conventional open adrenalectomy preferred to a laparoscopic procedure?

Minimally invasive procedures are gaining more popularity in the recent days. Open procedures require large incisions to allow accurate dissection and are therefore associated with long recovery times. The absolute contraindication to laparoscopic adrenalectomy is the presence of malignancy or clinical/radiological characteristics of malignancy. In these cases a greater exposure and more aggressive surgery precludes laparoscopic surgery. Large tumours of >10 cm are also best excised by an open approach primarily because they are at a greater risk of being malignant but also because of technical considerations.

Amputation (below knee)

1 What are the indications for limb amputation? Which is the commonest in the UK?

- Lower limb ischaemia secondary to atherosclerosis and/or diabetes is by far the commonest indication for amputation in the UK
- Trauma which is the commonest indication in the Third World
- Infection
- Malignancy
- Congenital deformity

2 What types of lower limb amputation do you know?

- Hip disarticulation or hindquarter amputation
- Transfemoral or above knee amputation (AKA)
- Through knee amputation
- Transtibial or below knee amputation (BKA)
- Through ankle or Syme's amputation
- Partial foot amputations

3 What pre-operative measures should be taken?

This is an entirely multidisciplinary process. All the members of the team (physiotherapy, occupational therapy (OT), rehabilitation specialist, prosthetic specialist, nursing staff, psychologists as well as the surgeon) must be involved and if possible meet the patient prior to surgery.

The level of amputation must be decided upon. This depends on the patients "rehabilitation potential", degree of tissue compromise, and severity and pattern of the vascular disease.

Finally a careful anaesthetic assessment is made, bearing in mind that these patients may have atherosclerosis affecting their renal, coronary and cerebral vasculture as well as other co-morbid factors such as hypertension and diabetes. They may even be heavy smokers with associated pulmonary compromise.

10

4 Name two common techniques used for a BKA

1 Long posterior flap (the Burgess and Romano technique)
2 Skew flap

5 How do you perform a BKA?

Position This is supine with the affected leg in a knee-flexed position.

Incision The preferred level is 10–14 cm below the tibial tuberosity. This skin incision is marked such that a long posterior skin flap is obtained. This must be at least twice as long posteriorly as it is anteriorly.

Procedure The skin incision is made through skin, subcutaneous fat and the muscles of the anterolateral compartments. All vessels are identified and ligated prior to division. All the nerves are cut under tension. The tibia and fibula are then sawed and bevelled smooth. The fibula can be shortened to a higher level than the site of the tibial transection by about 2–3 cm. The posterior compartment is then attended to. The flap is fashioned by thinning the gastrocnemius muscle. The soleus is excised and is not normally included with the flap as it can increase the bulk of the stump.

Closure The flap is closed after achieving haemostasis. Interrupted non-absorbable sutures are preferred.

6 What are the complications that are specific to a BKA?

- Early
  - Stump haematoma
  - Infection
  - Flap necrosis (may necessitate revision to a higher amputation level)
- Late
  - Painful neuromas
  - Infection
  - Bony erosion and stump ulceration
  - Pain and phantom pain
  - Ill-fitting prosthesis due to poorly fashioned stumps or stump atrophy
  - Psychological problems
  - Knee-joint contractures

7 What contraindications are there to a BKA?

- Poor mobility and the possibility of wheel-chair dependence. The BKA patient is prone to developing pressure sores

in this situation an AKA may be a more suitable procedure.
- A stump <5 cm, which will make fitting of the prosthesis difficult.
- Fixed flexion deformity of the knee.

Anorectal abscesses, fistulae and pilonidal sinus

1 Where do anorectal abscesses occur?

These abscess are usually caused by an infection in one of the anal glands in the intersphincteric space. As the infection worsens, there is the spread of pus, which may track to the skin causing a perianal abscess (most common), laterally through puborectalis causing an ischiorectal abscess, or more internally causing a supralevator abscess.

2 What are other causes of anorectal abscess?

Those not related to the anal glands and these are:

- Submucosal abscess from infected haemorrhoids or fissures
- Subcutaneous from an infected hair follicle

3 What is the usual organism responsible?

Gram-positive *Staphylococcus aureus* is the most common organism although occasionally bowel flora will cause an infection. If bowel flora is present there is a higher proportion of associated fistulae.

4 What is the surgical treatment?

Incision and drainage of the abscess under general anaesthetic is the treatment of choice.

5 How would you perform an incision and drainage of an anorectal abscess?

Pre-operatively The patient should be appropriately consented. There is no specific requirement for antibiotics unless the patient has cellulitis or is immunocompromised.

Position This is supine and in the lithotomy position. Rectal examination is then performed (proctoscopy/sigmoidoscopy) to search for an internal discharge or fistula opening (it is important not to probe in this acute setting as there is a risk of forming a fistula).

Incision A cruciate incision is made over the abscess at the point of maximal fluctuance.

Procedure A pus swab taken and sent for microscopy and sensitivities. The pus is drained out and loculations are broken down with a finger. Curettage is then performed to the wall of the abscess and any necrotic tissue is excised. Haemostasis is ensured to leave no major bleeding points. A washout with 0.5% hydrogen peroxide or saline is performed.

Packing and closure The cavity is normally lightly packed with a saline- or sterile-soaked gauze swab to prevent haematoma formation. The incision is left open to drain any remaining pus and allows secondary intention healing via granulation.

6 How are anal fistulae classified?

They may be split according to their relations with the anal sphincters:

- Intersphincteric
- Transsphincteric
- Suprasphincteric
- Extrasphincteric

They can also be described as high or low.

7 What is Goodsall's law?

This is a law, which predicts where the internal opening of the fistulae lies in relation to their external opening. For openings anterior to the transverse anal line, the fistula normally runs radially into the anal canal. For openings posterior to this line the track is in a semi-linear curve and opens into the anal lumen in the midline posteriorly (see diagram).

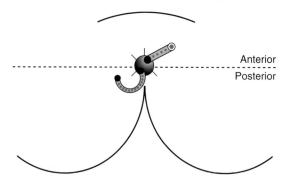

Anterior

Posterior

Anal fistulae
Anterior to line track radially
Posterior to line track in crescent

8 What are the treatment aims?

The aim is to achieve complete healing without compromising the anal sphincteric function.

9 Describe a fistulotomy

The operation should be performed following an MRI scan if uncertain about the tract anatomy, and ideally by an experienced colorectal surgeon.

Position Lithotomy.

Procedure Openings below the dentate line are usually safe to proceed. The external fistula is probed, and the track is curetted and laid open with a blade. If it is a high fistula then a loose Seton is placed which acts as a drainage Seton. This may be left long term, or it may be necessary to proceed with further more complex secondary surgical procedure at a later date.

10 What is a pilonidal sinus?

This is a chronic inflammatory condition describing the presence of at least one or more sinuses in the natal cleft, which contain debris and hair. It is secondary to hair follicle enlargement and subsequent ingrown hair accumulating in the cavity. It is more common in "hairy males".

The condition usually presents following abscess formation and is treated *acutely* in the manner mentioned above for abscesses.

As a later secondary procedure the pilonidal sinus is excised. The wound may then be closed primarily or left open to heal by granulation.

Appendicectomy

1 What is the differential diagnosis of acute appendicitis?

- Gastrointestinal
  - Acute cholecystitis
  - Mesenteric adenitis
  - Terminal ileitis
  - Diverticulitis
  - Carcinoid tumour
  - Meckel's diverticulum
- Gynaecological
  - Ectopic pregnancy
  - Torted ovarian cyst
  - Pelvic inflammatory disease
  - Mittelschmerz pain
- Genito-urological
  - Testicular torsion
  - Ureteric colic
  - Pyelonephritis
- Others
  - Diabetic ketoacidosis
  - Shingles
  - Porphyria

2 What is a Meckel's diverticulum?

This is a remnant of the vitelline duct. It occurs in 2% of the population; it may be 2 cm long and sited 2 feet proximal to the ileocaecal valve on the antimesenteric border of the ileum.

3 What is the blood supply to the appendix?

The appendicular artery supplies the appendix. This is a branch of the ileocolic artery arising from the superior mesenteric artery. It runs in the appendix mesentery.

4 What are the various anatomical positions of the appendix?

- 75%:Retrocolic and retrocaecal
- 20%:Subcaecal and pelvic
- 5%:Pre-ileal and retro-ileal

5 What is McBurney's point?

This is the surface marking of the base of the appendix and is sited at a point two-thirds of the way down a line drawn from the umbilicus to the anterior, superior iliac spine. It is the most tender spot on examination of a patient with appendicitis and a useful landmark in planning the site of the incision when performing an appendicectomy.

6 What pre-operative measures should be taken for an appendicectomy?

The patient should be adequately rehydrated and intravenous broad-spectrum antibiotics should be given if there is evidence of perforation (e.g. Cefotaxime and Metronidazole). The patient should be consented and in the elderly patient forewarned of the possibility of a conversion to a laparotomy.

7 How do you perform an appendicectomy?

Position This is supine with the surgeon standing to the patient's right. The abdomen is prepared as for a laparotomy.

Incision The incision may be a Gridiron (muscle splitting at McBurney's point) or a Lanz incision that may give a better cosmetic result (see diagram).

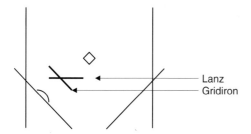

Lanz
Gridiron

The layers traversed are:

Skin
Subcutaneous fat
Scarpa's fascia
External oblique aponeurosis
Internal oblique
Transversus abdominus
Transversalis fascia
Pre-peritoneal fat
Parietal peritoneum

All muscles are split in the direction of their fibres.

Procedure The peritoneum is opened and a sample of fluid is swabbed and sent to microbiology. The caecum is gently drawn out of the incision and its taeniae coli are followed until they meet at the base of the appendix. It may be necessary to divide adhesions to mobilise the caecum.

The meso-appendix is clamped and divided with ligation of its vessels. The appendicular base is then crushed, ligated and divided. The appendix is removed and sent to histology. The stump may be buried or left everted. If there is free peritoneal fluid present lavage should be performed. A drain may be inserted in the presence of pus.

Closure The abdominal wall is closed in layers.

8 What are the complications of an appendicectomy?

- Immediate
  - Haemorrhage
- Early
  - Wound and pelvic infection
  - Peritonitis
  - Post-operative ileus
- Late
  - Adhesions leading to bowel obstruction

6

Principles of bowel anastomosis

1 What are the layers of the bowel wall? (See diagram)

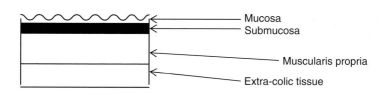

2 What factors are important in bowel anastomotic healing?

- Patient factors
  - Co-morbidity (poorer healing in the immunocompromised or diabetics)
  - Poor nutritional status
  - Smoking
- Surgical technique
  - Accurate apposition of bowel ends
  - Lack of tension
  - Ensuring a good blood supply to both bowel ends

- Peri-operative considerations
  - Intraperitoneal sepsis (therefore prescribing peri-operative antibiotics)
  - Ensuring that there is no obstruction distal to the anastomosis
  - Hypotension

3 What is the "gold standard" method of bowel anastomosis?

Most surgeons adopt an interrupted single-layer serosubmucosal technique as the gold standard using an absorbable suture.

4 What other methods are used in bowel anastomosis?

- Single layer continuous
- Double layer
- Stapled
- Sutureless (e.g. tissue glue and compression rings)

5 What are the advantages and disadvantages of the stapled technique?

- Advantages
  - Quicker
  - Easier in less accessible areas (e.g. in abdomino-perineal resections of the rectum)
  - Safer to the surgeon
- Disadvantages
  - Malposition of the staple or malfunction of the device cannot easily be redeemed with replacement hand-sewn sutures.
  - The device and staples are more expensive than sutures.
  - Has an increase frequency of anastomotic stricture formation.

Breast surgery

1 When should a mastectomy be performed in preference to breast conserving surgery?

A mastectomy is preferred to breast conserving procedures in:

- Multifocal or widespread disease
- Breast cancer in men
- Treatment of recurrence after breast conservation surgery.

Relative indications include:

- A large tumour in a small breast
- Tumour close to the nipple.

2 What is the arterial blood supply to the breast?

Branches from the anterior intercostal arteries (internal thoracic artery) supply the medial part of the breast.

Laterally a network of anastomosis from branches of the axillary artery provide the blood supply. These include the lateral thoracic artery, pectoral branch of the thoracoacromial artery and the superior thoracic artery.

3 What different forms of mastectomy do you know? What do they involve?

- *Simple mastectomy*: This refers to the excision of the whole breast, its axillary tail, the nipple and any involved overlying skin but preserving the pectoralis fascia. Axillary surgery is not performed.
- *Radical mastectomy*: This is the excision of the entire breast tissue, pectoralis major and minor muscles, and a complete axillary clearance.
- *Patey radical mastectomy*: In this procedure pectoralis major muscle is spared but pectoralis minor is removed to allow a complete axillary clearance.

4 What different types of axillary surgery do you know?

- *Axillary lymph node sampling*: This refers to the removal of at least four prominent axillary lymph nodes. If the nodes are positive then further treatment in the form of radiotherapy or axillary clearance is offered to the patient.
- *Axillary clearance*: This refers to the complete clearance of the axillary lymph nodes and is associated with significant morbidity.
- *Sentinel node biopsy*: The sentinel node(s) is/are the first node(s) that the tumour is drained by. This is identified, using radioisotope labelling, and biopsies are taken. If negative, no further axillary procedure is indicated.

5 What are the three levels of axillary lymph nodes?

- *Level I*: Nodes inferior to pectoralis minor muscle
- *Level II*: Nodes posterior to pectoralis minor muscle
- *Level III*: Nodes superior to pectoralis minor muscle

6 How do you perform a simple mastectomy?

Pre-operatively The side is marked. If the tumour is not easily palpable it is localised using a hooked wire radiologically. Psychological preparation with a multidisciplinary team approach is of utmost importance.

Position The patient is placed supine with the arm supported on an arm board. Routine preparation and draping is performed.

Incision An elliptical incision is made above and below the nipple, incorporating the tumour.

Procedure Skin flaps are carefully raised medially as far as the lateral edge of the sternum and laterally into the axilla. Dissection is continued superiorly as far as the clavicular head of pectoralis major and inferiorly to the base of the breast. The breast tissue is then removed from the underlying fascia. Medially the branches of the internal thoracic artery (see Question 2 above) and laterally those from the axillary artery are ligated. Care is taken to avoid damage to the axillary vein and the long thoracic nerve. The tail of the breast is also removed.

Closure Two suction drains are placed and the skin defect is closed in a single layer.

7 List some of the specific complications of breast surgery

- Immediate
  - Haemorrhage
- Early
  - Infection
  - Skin flap necrosis
  - Seroma

- Late
  - Lymphoedema (secondary to axillary lymph node surgery or damage to the axillary vein)
  - Damage to the long thoracic nerve (winging of scapula)
  - Psychological problems
  - Recurrence

8 Name two methods commonly used in breast reconstruction following mastectomy

1 Subpectoral tissue expansion which can be later replaced by a silicone implant.
2 Myocutaneous flaps for example latissimus dorsi flap or transverse rectus abdominus myocutaneous (TRAM) flap.

Carotid endarterectomy

1 What are the indications for a carotid endarterectomy?

Carotid endarterectomy is indicated in symptomatic patients with symptoms suggestive of ischaemia in the carotid territory (TIA or Amaurosis Fugax) who have a major degree of carotid stenosis (between 70% and 99%). This is based on results from the European Carotid Surgery Trial (ECST) and the North American Symptomatic Carotid Endarterectomy Trial (NASCET). Patients who have symptoms suggesting insufficiency of the vertebro-basilar circulation are not included.

There is currently a randomised clinical trial, which is looking at asymptomatic patients with carotid stenosis (the Asymptomatic Carotid Surgery Trial).

2 What are the clinical presentations of ischaemia of the carotid and the vertebro-basilar circulations?

- *Carotid*: contralateral hemiparesis, hemianopia, hemisensory disturbances as well as dysphasia (dominant hemisphere) or visuospatial apraxias.

- *Vertebrobasilar*: Vertigo, diplopia, dysphagia, dysphonia, nausea, vomiting or ataxia

3 What pre-operative measures should be taken?

- To establish the diagnosis and grade the stenosis, duplex scanning is the investigation of choice in most centres. Patients were previously investigated using IADSA; but this itself carries a 1–2% risk of stroke. Some centres are now using magnetic resonance angiography (MRA) as an alternative. The patient will also require a CT scan of the brain to establish pre-operative infarcted areas.
- Anaesthetic assessment and informed consent.
- The patient should have an intravenous line and an arterial line in situ.
- The side should be marked.

4 How do you perform a carotid endarterectomy?

Position The patient is placed supine with the shoulders elevated on a cushion to extend the neck. The head should be turned away. The skin should be prepared from the neck to the thorax.

Incision An anterior sternocleidomastoid incision should be made at the level of the hyoid.

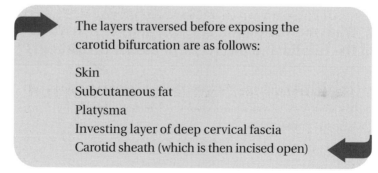

The layers traversed before exposing the carotid bifurcation are as follows:

Skin
Subcutaneous fat
Platysma
Investing layer of deep cervical fascia
Carotid sheath (which is then incised open)

Procedure Slings are placed around the common, internal and external carotid arteries. The vessels are heparinised. The vessels are occluded (start the stop-watch measuring carotid occlusion time). An arteriotomy is performed followed by the endarterectomy. If a shunt is needed it is placed above and below the occlusion at this stage.

Closure Close the arteriotomy. The clamps are then released releasing the distal clamp of the internal carotid last. Closure is in layers.

5 What vertebral level does the carotid bifurcation correspond to and what is its surface marking?

The carotid bifurcation is at the level of the fourth cervical vertebrae, which may be indicated by a point under the anterior border of the sternocleidmastoid (SCM) muscle at the upper edge of the thyroid cartilage.

6 During surgery what features will help distinguish the external from the internal carotid artery?

- The origin of the ECA is anteromedial to the origin of the ICA.
- The ICA has no branches outside the skull.
- The carotid sinus may be visible at the origin of the ICA as a subtle dilatation.

7 Which nerves are at risk during carotid surgery?

- Vagus nerve
- Glossopharyngeal nerve
- Hypoglossal nerve

- Ansa cervicalis
- External laryngeal nerve

8 What other complications of carotid endarterectomy do you know?

The risk of early stroke varies between 5% and 7% in the ECST and NASCET trials. The risk of mortality is <2%.

9 What techniques are available for monitoring cerebral function during carotid endarterectomy?

- Awake monitoring under local anaesthesia
- Stump pressure measurement. A shunt is required if the internal carotid artery pressure is less than a third of radial artery pressure
- Transcranial Doppler
- EEG
- Monitoring transcranial oxygen pressures using near infrared spectroscopy

9

················

Carpal tunnel decompression

1 What is carpal tunnel syndrome (CTS)?

CTS is defined as median nerve compression neuropathy at the carpal tunnel. This is a fibro-osseous canal, the roof of which is formed by the flexor retinaculum and the floor by the carpal bones and their joining ligaments.

2 List some of the causes of this condition

Most cases are idiopathic, however fluid retention as seen in pregnancy can cause the syndrome. Other associated conditions include: rheumatoid arthritis, diabetes, hypothyroidism, acromegaly, amyloid, wrist ganglions and fractures.

3 What non-surgical options are there in the treatment of CTS?

Splinting, in particular at nighttime, or injection of corticosteroids into the carpal tunnel.

4 How do you perform a carpal tunnel decompression (CTD)?

Pre-operatively The diagnosis is confirmed clinically and/or with nerve conduction studies. Informed consent is taken, explaining the risks and benefits of the procedure. A choice of local anaesthetic versus general anaesthetic depends on patient's condition and surgeon preference. A tourniquet may be used.

Position This is supine with the affected arm on a supporting table. The hand and forearm are then prepared and draped.

Procedure A 4–6-cm palmar *incision* is made ulnar to the mid-line to avoid damage to the sensory palmar branch of the median nerve. The proximal extent will be the distal crease of the wrist. This is made through skin, subcutaneous fat and palmar/forearm fascia. Flexor retinaculum is then identified and incised along the line of the incision (directing the distal extension of this incision in an ulnar direction to avoid the recurrent motor branch of the median nerve). The median nerve may be protected using a Macdonald retractor.

Closure The skin closure is then undertaken after adequate haemostasis is achieved.

5 What structures pass under the flexor retinaculum?

- Tendons of flexor digitorium superficialis
- Median nerve
- Tendons of flexor digitorium profundus
- Tendon of flexor pollicis longus

6 What structures maybe at risk in a CTD?

- Sensory palmar branch of the median nerve that supplies an area of skin overlying the thenar eminence
- Recurrent motor branch of the median nerve that provides motor supply to the thenar muscles
- The median nerve
- Superficial palmar arterial arch

7 What other complications will you mention to the patient during consent?

Infection at the wound site, the possible failure of surgical treatment and the need for revision surgery.

33

10

....

Central venous cannulation

1 List some of the indications for a central venous cannula

- Measurement of right-heart filling pressure to guide fluid balance
- Administration of parenteral nutrition
- Administration of drugs that should be administered via a central vein (e.g. inotropes)
- Access for introduction of pulmonary artery catheter, pacing wires, etc.
- Establishing intravenous access if peripheral access is not possible

2 What different routes can be chosen for central vein access?

- Internal jugular vein
- Subclavian vein (this can be infra or supracalvicular)
- Femoral vein
- Peripheral veins (PICC lines)

3 Describe the course and relationships of the subclavian vein

The axillary vein becomes the subclavian vein at the level of the outer border of the first rib. It then proceeds medially, superior to the first rib and anterior to the scalenus anterior muscle. It remains behinds the clavicle and in close proximity to the dome of the pleura.

4 Describe the course and the relationships of the internal jugular vein

The internal jugular vein exits the base of the skull through the jugular foramen that corresponds to a point approximately one finger's breadth behind the lobe of the ear. It descends vertically and in its lower third lies behind the sternocleidomastoid muscle. It terminates at the medial end of the clavicle. This vein lies within the carotid sheath and in close proximity to the common carotid artery and the vagus nerve. The lower end of the internal jugular lies at the space between the sternal and clavicular heads of the sternocleidomastoid.

5 Describe the technique of inserting a central line via the subclavian route

Position This procedure can be performed under local anaesthetic. The patient is placed in a 30-degree head down or Trendelenburg position. The area is cleaned and draped under a strict aseptic technique and the local anaesthetic infiltrated. A left-sided approach is preferred.

Procedure The needle entry point is the inferior surface of the midpoint of the clavicle at the level of its anterior bow. The needle is advance horizontally towards the sternal notch.

The following layers are traversed:

Skin

Subcutaneous fat

Fascia

Pectoralis major muscle

Subclavius muscle

Subclavian vein

Venous entry is confirmed with the backflow of venous blood. The central line is then inserted using the Seldinger technique: the syringe is removed and the needle held in position for the guidewire to be inserted through it. With the guidewire in position the needle can be withdrawn. The entry point on the skin is dilated before the central line is inserted over the wire. *Note*: It is important to flush all lumens with saline, prior to insertion, to prevent air embolism.

Closure The line is secured to the skin using silk sutures and appropriate dressings applied. A chest radiograph must be obtained to confirm correct placement before the line is used.

6 Describe the technique of inserting a central line via the internal jugular route

Position is as for subclavian cannulation. The entry point is on the medial border of the sternocleidomastoid at the level of the thyroid cartilage. The course of the internal carotid is determined by palpating its pulsations. The needle is advanced parallel but lateral to it aiming towards the opposite nipple.

Recently National Institute for Clinical Excellence (NICE) has recommended ultrasound guidance to optimise the success rate of cannulations and minimise complications.

> The layers traversed are:
>
> Skin
> Subcutaneous fat
> Platysma
> Investing layer of cervical fascia
> Carotid sheath
> Internal jugular vein

Once venous entry is confirmed the central line is introduced using the Seldinger technique described above.

7 What are the possible complications of central venous cannulation?

- Infection
- Bleeding, which is worse if it is due to puncture of an artery that is in the proximity of the vein
- Air embolism
- Pneumothorax (more common with subclavian cannulation)
- Nerve injury (brachial plexus, phrenic, recurrent laryngeal, vagus)
- Injury to thoracic duct (chylothorax)
- Tracheal or endotracheal tube injury
- Cardiac arrhythmias

· · · · · · · · · · · · · · · · ·

11

Cholecystectomy (laparoscopic)

1 What are the contraindications to a laparoscopic cholecystectomy?

With increasing usage and experience in this technique, it is possible to perform this operation under most circumstances, however, relative contraindications include:

- Previous abdominal surgery or adhesions
- Clotting disorder
- Peritonitis
- Dilated bowel
- Morbid obesity
- Pregnancy

2 What are the advantages of laparoscopic surgery?

- Advantages to the patient
  - Less painful due to less tissue damage
  - Reduced hospital stay
  - Fewer adhesions
  - Fewer incisional herniae
  - Better cosmetic result

- Advantages to the surgeon
  - Fewer "Sharps" injuries
  - Less contact with blood
  - Easier in obese patients than open

3 What pre-operative measures should be taken before a laparoscopic cholecystectomy?

- Peri-operative antibiotics according to local policy (e.g. three doses of Cefotaxime and Metronidazole).
- The use of a nasogastric tube (NGT) to deflate the stomach and a urethral catheter to empty the bladder remains controversial.

4 Describe both the open and closed methods of creating a pneumoperitoneum

- *Open*: Dissection down through the linea alba is made via a subumbilical incision. The peritoneum is elevated with two clips and incised, allowing the blunt 10-mm trocar to be introduced into the peritoneal cavity. Carbon dioxide is then introduced into the peritoneal cavity (in an adult this amounts to 2–3 l with pressures not exceeding 15 mmHg).
- *Closed*: This uses a spring loaded Verres needle which is blindly introduced into the peritoneal cavity after manually elevating the anterior abdominal wall. Its use is no longer recommended since it has a high complication rate of causing damage to blood vessels and intra-abdominal organs.

5 What is Calot's triangle?

This triangle contains the cystic artery (which usually arises from the right hepatic artery). It is bounded superiorly by the caudate lobe of the liver; medially by the common hepatic duct and laterally by the cystic duct. This triangle is dissected out and the cystic artery identified and clipped before the gall bladder can be safely removed.

6 How do you perform a laparoscopic cholecystectomy?

Position This is supine with a head up tilt and rolled to the left. The patient is prepared and draped as for a laparotomy.

Incision A pneumoperitoneum is induced using one of the methods described above at the subumbilical site. Two to three further "stab" incisions are made under direct vision (with the camera inserted into the 10-mm cannula at the subumbilical site). These incisions are at the midline epigastrium, the right subcostal region at the midclavicular line and at the anterior axillary line.

Procedure Calot's triangle is identified (see above). The cystic duct and artery are ligated. An operative cholangiogram may then be performed to clearly define biliary anatomy, to visualise free flow into the duodenum and to identify unsuspected stones in the common bile duct (CBD). The gall bladder is then removed via the subumbilical site and sent for histological investigation.

Closure Absolute haemostasis must be ensured and the subumbilical port site is closed in layers. "Steri-strips" are applied to the stab incisions.

7 What are the specific complications of a laparoscopic cholecystectomy?

- Immediate
  - Haemorrhage (cystic artery damage)

- Excessive CO_2 insufflation splinting the diaphragm leading to inadequate oxygenation
- CBD damage (can cause hole or strictures)
- Early
  - Bile leak (occurs in 0.3%)
  - Wound infection
  - Post-operative ileus
  - Shoulder tip pain
- Late
  - Incisional hernia
  - Biliary stricture
  - Pancreatitis

12

· · · · · · · · · · · · · · · ·

Circumcision

1 What are the indications for a circumcision?

- Medical
  - Phimosis
  - Paraphimosis
  - Balanitis xerotica obliterans (BXO)
  - Delayed physiological phimosis
- Religious and social

2 What are the potential complications of a circumcision?

- Haemorrhage, which can be primary or secondary
- Infection
- Urethral injury
- Painful scars
- Reduction of sensation of the glans penis post-operatively

3 How do you perform a circumcision?

Position This is supine. A routine preparation and drape is performed. A penile block can be used to provide post-operative analgesia.

Incision and procedure The foreskin is grasped at the edge of its opening with artery forceps. Dorsal and ventral slits are made cutting through both the inner mucosa and the outer layer. The foreskin is then cut freehand around the coronal sulcus with scissors. A mucosal cuff is fashioned to allow closure.

Closure All bleeding points are identified and cauterised with bipolar diathermy before circumferential interrupted sutures are inserted. Local anaesthetic gel or Chloramphenicol ointment is used.

4 How do you manage a patient with early post-circumcision bleeding?

Most early haemorrhage is self-limiting and responds to pressure dressings, however if the bleeding has continued despite a normal clotting profile the patient needs to be returned to theatre for further diathermy or re-suturing. If a penile block was used in theatre, sutures can be applied at the bedside.

Colles' fracture (closed reduction of)

1 Who was Colles?

Abraham Colles, Irish surgeon and anatomist (1773–1843) described, amongst other things, fractures of the distal radius within 2.5 cm of the joint with dorsal displacement. He described this in the elderly, post-menopausal women and therefore distal radial fractures in other groups of patients are not, strictly speaking, Colles' fractures.

2 What are the five characteristic features of a Colles' fracture?

1 Dorsal displacement of the distal fragment
2 Dorsal angulation of the distal fragment
3 Radial displacement of the distal fragment
4 Shortening or impaction
5 Avulsion of the ulnar styloid process

3 What options of anaesthesia do you know for reduction of Colles' fractures?

- Haematoma block
- Biers block
- Axillary/brachial plexus blocks
- General anaesthesia

4 How do you reduce a Colles' fractures?

This aims to correct the deformities described in Question 2, after the appropriate anaesthesia is selected and informed consent is obtained.

- Disimpaction is the essential first stage. This is done by applying gentle but constant traction along the line of the forearm whilst an assistant is applying counter-traction with the elbow in 90 degrees of flexion.
- Manipulation is then undertaken by applying pressure to correct the dorsal displacement/angulation and radial deviation of the distal fragment. At times it is necessary to increase the deformity, to "unlock" the distal fragment, prior to manipulation.
- A Plaster of Paris "back slab" is then applied to maintain the reduction. This will also allow for any early swelling prior to completion of the cast. The position is in full pronation and slight ulnar deviation with the wrist in flexion.

A check radiograph is then obtained to confirm reduction. The plaster is completed after the first week.

5 What are the options for maintaining the reduction in distal radial fractures?

- Plaster cast
- K-wires

- Plates and screws
- External fixation
- A combination of above

6 What are the complications of distal radial fractures?

- Malunion which can result in long-term wrist pain and loss in function
- Non-union or delayed union
- Stiffness
- Carpal tunnel syndrome
- Osteoarthritis, OA (particularly in those fractures with intra-articular extension)
- Rupture of the extensor pollicis longus tendon
- Sudeck's atrophy (this is a form of reflex sympathetic dystrophy that may affect the hands after an injury)

14

················

Compound fractures

1 Why are compound fractures of significance?

A compound or open fracture is important as it signifies
a greater degree of soft-tissue damage that needs urgent
assessment and may require reconstructive surgery in the
future. A compound fracture has a much greater risk of
complications such as infection, delayed or non-union.

2 What is the initial management of a patient with a compound fracture?

Many patients with compound fractures also have significant
other injuries and maybe in shock. A thorough advanced
trauma life support assessment to identify and correct any
life-threatening injuries should be the first step. Other specific
measures include:

- Assessment and documentation of the wound. Ideally a
  photograph should be taken, the wound covered with a
  sterile dressing and left undisturbed until the patient is in
  theatre. A wound swab may be taken prior to dressing.
- Assessment and documentation of the neuro-vascular status
  of the limb.
- Intravenous prophylaxis antibiotics.

- Tetanus prophylaxis.
- Analgesia.
- Splintage of the affected limb (Thomas' splint, Plaster of Paris, etc.).
- Radiographs of the limb and the surrounding joints are obtained in two views.

3 Describe Gustilo's classification of open fractures

- *Type I* Small, clean, puncture wound (<1 cm) as a result of a low energy injury with little soft-tissue damage
- *Type II* The wound is >1 cm but again the degree of soft-tissue damage is low
- *Type III* These are as the result of high-energy trauma with extensive soft-tissue damage and contamination:
  - *Type IIIA* adequate bony cover can be achieved
  - *Type IIIB* there is comminution, periosteal stripping and bone loss and the wound is heavily contaminated
  - *Type IIIC* there is associated neuro-vascular compromise.

4 What are the principles of managing open fractures when in theatre?

- Wound debridement – excision of all devitalised tissue
- Wound extension to allow adequate visualisation of the wound and the fracture
- Irrigation with large amounts of sterile saline (solution to pollution is dilution) up to 12 l of saline may be used for long bone fractures
- Stabilisation of the fracture (external fixation, intramedullary (IM) nails, etc.)
- Wound cover – wounds must be left open and loosely packed with a sterile dressing
- Secondary look and debridement after 48 hours

5 Which antibiotics would you choose to give to a patient with an open fracture?

In most instances a second generation Cephalosporin given for the first 48 hours should suffice. However, for more severe injuries and if the wound is heavily contaminated Gram-negative prophylaxis such as an aminoglycoside (Gentamicin) as well as Metronidazole should be considered.

If there is a risk of clostridial infection intravenous Penicillin should also be given.

6 What tetanus prophylaxis would you chose to give?

The choice is between the vaccine (toxoid) and tetanus human immunoglobulin (Ig).

	Wound type	
Immune status	Clean	Tetanus prone
Last of 3-dose course, or a single reinforcing dose given WITHIN last 10 years	Nil	Nil (if particularly contaminated then human tetanus Ig may be given)
Last of 3-dose course or a single reinforcing dose MORE than 10 years ago	Single-dose tetanus toxoid	Single-dose tetanus toxoid + human tetanus Ig
Not immunised	Full 3-dose course of tetanus vaccination	Full 3-dose course + human tetanus Ig

15

Dupuytren's contracture release

1 What is Dupuytren's disease?

This is a nodular thickening of the palmar aponeurosis leading to flexion contractures of the fingers at the metacarpophalangeal joint (MCPJ) and/or proximal interphalangeal joint (PIPJ) of the fingers. The ring and little fingers are most commonly affected. The condition has a higher prevalence in people from northern European descent.

2 What conditions are associated with Dupuytren's disease?

This condition is mainly idiopathic and familial (autosomal dominant), however there is a high incidence in epileptics on phenytoin and is also known to be associated with diabetes, alcoholic cirrhosis, AIDS and pulmonary tuberculosis.

3 What other associated clinical manifestations of Dupuytren's disease do you know?

- Thickenings on the dorsum of the fingers (Garrod's pads)
- Thickening of the plantar fascia of the feet

- Thickening and fibrosis of the corpous cavernosum of the penis (Peyronie's disease)

4 What are the surgical options in treating the condition?

- *Fasciotomy*: Release of the contracture without excising the thickened bands.
- *Fasciectomy*: Excision of all diseased bands contributing to the deformity.
- *Dermatofasciectomy*: As above with the addition of a full-thickness skin graft to an excised skin defect.
- *Amputation*: May be necessary in severe recurrent disease.

5 Briefly discuss how you would perform a Dupuytren's excision

Position This is supine with the affected arm on a supporting table. The hand and forearm are then prepared and draped. The arm is exsanguinated and a tourniquet is applied.

Incision: A zigzag or Brunner incision is made from midpalm proximal to the contracture and into the finger. Skin flaps are then carefully raised.

Procedure This involves careful identification and protection of both the digital neuro-vascular bundles of the affected digit before excising as much Dupuytren's tissue as possible.

Closure Direct closure may be possible, however, advancement flaps in the form of Y–V-flaps or Z-plasties may be required. In some cases a full-thickness skin graft taken from the volar forearm skin may be necessary.

6 What specific risks of surgery would you explain to your patient during the consent process?

- Damage to the digital neuro-vascular bundles of the fingers with sensory abnormality of the affected finger.
- Risk of recurrence and need for revision surgery.
- Small but serious risk of a digital amputation, especially in recurrent surgery.

7 Who was Dupuytren?

Baron Guillaume Dupuytren was born in 1777 and died in 1835 in Paris. He was the first to publish on the contracture of the palmar fascia in a medical journal (Permanent retraction of the fingers, produced by affection of the palmar fascia. *Lancet*, London, 1833–1834, 2: 222–225). However the condition had previously been described by Sir Astley Cooper, and also mentioned by the Swiss physician Felix Platter (1536–1614).

16

Dynamic hip screw

1 How does one classify femoral neck fractures on the basis of their anatomy? How does this influence management?

These can be divided into *intra-capsular* or *extra-capsular* fractures with respect to their relationship to the capsule of the hip joint. Intra-capsular fractures have a high risk of avascular necrosis (AVN) of the femoral head and these fractures are treated with a femoral head replacement in most cases. Extra-capsular fractures are internally fixed with devices such as the dynamic hip screw (DHS) or trochanteric nails.

2 What is the anatomical reason for AVN in intra-capsular fractures?

The greater part of the blood supply to the femoral head is via the retinacular vessels which in turn arise from the anastomosis of the medial and lateral circumflex femoral arteries. These retinacular vessels are closely related to the capsule and may be interrupted in cases of intra-capsular fractures, rendering the femoral head ischaemic.

3 What are the options in treating intra-capsular femoral neck fractures?

- Trial of conservative management with early mobilisation under supervision.
- Hemiarthroplasty (e.g. cemented, uncemented, bipolar)
- Internal fixation (e.g. DHS, cannulated screws)
- Total hip arthroplasty

4 In what circumstances would an intra-capsular fracture be treated with an internal fixation device?

In these fractures there is a high risk of AVN of the femoral head and femoral head replacement (hemiarthroplasty or THR) is a preferred mode of treatment. However in young patients (<65 years old) and/or those with undisplaced fractures (and therefore with little disruption of retinacular vessels) internal fixation may be contemplated.

5 How do you perform internal fixation of a femoral neck fracture using the DHS?

Pre-operatively The medical condition of the patient is optimised. Consent is obtained, the side is marked and intravenous antibiotics are given at induction and for 24 hours post-operatively.

Position This is supine on a traction table. The fracture is reduced closed, usually by maintaining traction and internal rotation. The unaffected hip is flexed and abducted to allow access for an image intensifier.

Approach A lateral incision is made, starting from just below the tip of the greater trochanter and along the line of the femoral shaft.

> The layers traversed are:
>
> Skin
> Subcutaneous fat
> Fascia lata
> Vastus lateralis (which is split by blunt dissection)
> Periosteum

Procedure After ensuring reduction has been maintained, a guidewire is passed into the centre of the femoral head and its position is checked in the anteroposterior (AP) and lateral planes using image intensification. The screw length is measured. The bone is then reamed over the guidewire using the triple-reamer. The bone is then tapped and the appropriate screw inserted. The guidewire can then be removed. Finally, the DHS plate is fixed onto the femoral shaft, sliding over the screw.

Closure This is in layers after achieving haemostasis.

6 What are the complications of a DHS?

- General complications include myocardial infarction, stroke, pneumonia, thrombosis, urinary tract infections and pressure sores. These in the compromised elderly can result in death.
- Specific complications include wound infection, wound dehiscence, deep infection, delayed union, non-union and device failure (with screw or plate fracture; or "cutting out" of the screw).

59

17

······················

Fasciotomy for compartment syndrome

1 What is compartment syndrome?

Compartment syndrome is an abnormal elevation of the hydrostatic pressure within a closed fascial compartment. This will lead to cell death, oedema and ultimately will result in a further rise in pressure. This is a vicious cycle, which, if left untreated can rapidly lead to ischaemia and death of the affected compartment (see diagram).

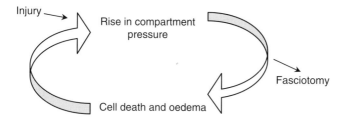

Injury → Rise in compartment pressure → Fasciotomy → Cell death and oedema

2 What are the clinical features of compartment syndrome?

- Pain, which is out of proportion to what is expected from the injury (the most important feature).

- Pain on passive stretch of the tendons/muscles that traverse the affected compartment.
- Affected compartments will be tense and swollen.
- Neuro-vascular compromise is a late feature.

3 What is a normal compartment pressure?

This is compared to the patient's diastolic blood pressure. The difference between the compartment pressure and the diastolic blood pressure (delta pressure) must be >30 mmHg for it to be considered normal. For example a compartment pressure of 28 mmHg in a patient with a BP of 100/50 mmHg is considered elevated (delta pressure is 22 mmHg).

4 When is compartmental pressure monitoring indicated?

Compartment syndrome is a clinical diagnosis and treatment should not be delayed by pressure monitoring. In cases where the clinical findings are inconclusive or the patient is unable to communicate (due to a reduced conscious level, learning disability, etc.) then pressure monitoring can be a helpful adjunct to clinical evaluation.

5 Name the compartments of the lower leg and list their contents

- *Anterior compartment*: Tibialis anterior, extensor hallucis longus, extensor digitorium longus, peroneus tertius, anterior tibial artery and the deep peroneal nerve.
- *Lateral compartment*: Peroneus longus, peroneus brevis, peroneal artery and the superficial peroneal nerve.

- *Posterior (superficial)*: Gastrocnemius, soleus and plantaris.
- *Posterior (deep)*: Tibialis posterior, flexor digitorium longus, flexor hallucis longus, posterior tibial artery and the posterior tibial nerve.

6 What is the technique for fasciotomy of the leg?

One technique is to perform a double-incision fasciotomy.

Pre-operatively The diagnosis is confirmed clinically. The patient is consented and in particular warned of large unsightly scars and the likelihood of multiple visits to the operating theatre for wound closures.

Position Patient is placed supine a tourniquet must not be used as this will cause a further rise in the compartment pressures.

Incision The first is halfway between the shaft of the fibula and the crest of the tibia (used to decompress the anterior and the lateral compartments); the second is two fingerbreadths posterior to the posterior margin of the tibia (used to decompress the deep and superficial posterior compartments).

Procedure All four of the fascial compartments are adequately decompressed.

Closure This is not performed. The wounds are packed and left open.

7 What are the compartments of the thigh?

Three compartments:
1 Anterior (quadriceps)
2 Posterior (hamstrings)
3 Medial (adductors)

63

8 What are the compartments of the forearm?

Three compartments:
1 Anterior, that can be further subdivided into deep and superficial compartments containing the deep and superficial flexors, respectively.
2 Posterior, containing the extensors.
3 The "mobile wad" compartment (containing brachioradialis and extensor carpi radialis longus and brevis).

18

Femoral embolectomy

1 What are the indications for a femoral embolectomy?

A femoral embolectomy is indicated for acute lower limb ischaemia due to suspected embolisation. This can be determined by careful history taking (no prior signs or symptoms of peripheral vascular disease, but perhaps with a history of atrial fibrillation, chest pain or palpitations) coupled with an urgent arteriogram.

2 What pre-operative measures should be taken?

- The patient should be adequately resuscitated with intravenous fluids and oxygen.
- The patient should receive Aspirin.
- The patient should receive an intravenous bolus of Heparin (e.g. 10,000 IU) followed by an infusion (10,000 IU 6 hourly) to prevent clot propagation.
- The patient should have 4 units of blood cross-matched.
- The patient's groin should be shaved and marked.
- Consider whether the patient is fit for a general or local anaesthetic.

3 How do you perform a femoral embolectomy?

Position This is supine with skin preparation of the abdomen, both groins and both thighs.

Incision A vertical incision over the femoral artery (at the midinguinal point).

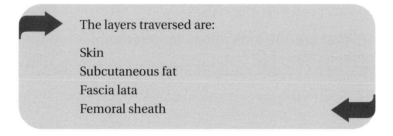

The layers traversed are:

Skin
Subcutaneous fat
Fascia lata
Femoral sheath

Procedure Expose the common femoral and its superficial and profunda branches. Assess for a pulse and place silastic rings around the vessels to control the flow.

Perform an arteriotomy and remove any clot. Insert a Fogarty catheter and inflate (proximally first and then distally).

Closure Close with 4/0 Prolene and then check for distal pulses. Closure is in layers.

4 What are the complications specific to a femoral embolectomy?

- Immediate
  - Haemorrhage
- Early
  - Revascularisation can lead to compartment syndrome (a prophylactic fasciotomy may be performed at the time of surgery)

- Reperfusion shock (due to the release of potassium, toxic metabolites and myoglobin)
- Acute tubular necrosis (due to the release of myoglobin from damaged muscle leading to myoglobinuria)
- Late
  - Recurrent thrombosis (especially if the original pathology was misdiagnosed as an embolus instead of thrombosis)

5 What is a Fogarty catheter?

Invented in 1963 by Thomas Fogarty, the Fogarty catheter is a plastic, flexible catheter with a balloon at its distal end. This is inflated with a syringe at its proximal end. It is then withdrawn to remove the clot.

6 What is the surface marking of the femoral artery?

The femoral artery runs along the proximal two-thirds of a line drawn from the midinguinal point (a point midway between the pubic symphysis and the anterior superior iliac spine) to the adductor tubercle.

67

19

················

Femoral hernia repair

1 Where does a femoral hernia occur?

This occurs through the femoral ring and into the femoral canal.

2 Name the borders of the femoral ring and the contents of the femoral canal

The femoral ring borders are:

Medial	Lacunar ligament
Lateral	Femoral vein
Anterior	Inguinal ligament
Posterior	Pectineal ligament and superior pubic ramus

It is important that three out of the four borders are rigid and so there is little room for expansion of hernial contents and the consequence of this is that strangulation is more common (compared to inguinal hernias). The femoral canal is approximately 1.5 cm long and contains lymph nodes (of Cloquet), which drain the penis or clitoris, connective tissue and lymph vessels.

3 Why are femoral herniae more common in women?

These are more common in women because the inguinal ligament makes a more oblique angle onto the pubis in females. The increased intra-abdominal pressure during pregnancy stretches the transversalis fascia and may also be a contributing factor.

4 What usually herniates into the femoral canal?

It is normally the mesentry that herniates, although it also may contain small bowel. In 30% of strangulated herniae there may be a functional obstruction with only a part of the lumen obstructed. This is known as a "Richter's hernia". Due to the high risk of strangulation, surgery is always recommended.

5 How do you differentiate between inguinal and femoral herniae?

This can be difficult:

Anatomically A femoral hernia is below and medial to the pubic tubercle.

Clinically A femoral hernia is usually small, painful and irreducible; there is usually no cough impulse or audible bowel sound.

6 What surgical options do you know for the repair of a femoral hernia?

There are three approaches to the hernia:
1 Low or crural approach (Lockwood) – used for elective and acute cases

2 Extra-peritoneal (modified McEvedy)
3 High or inguinal approach (Lothestein) – interferes with
   inguinal canal

Each technique has the principle of dissection of the sac with
reduction of its contents, followed by ligation of the sac and
closure between the inguinal and pectineal ligaments. The most
commonly used and simplest approach is the crural approach
although this does not allow easy visualisation of strangulated
bowel.

7 How do you perform a repair of a strangulated femoral hernia?

Pre-operatively General anaesthetic and antibiotics are given
(e.g. a Cephalosporin and Metronidazole).

Position This is supine with the groin and abdomen prepared
and draped.

Incision A 6-cm transverse incision is made directly over the
hernia (usually 2 cm below inguinal ligament).

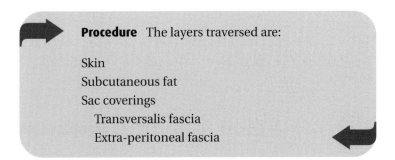

Procedure The layers traversed are:

Skin
Subcutaneous fat
Sac coverings
   Transversalis fascia
   Extra-peritoneal fascia

The sac is identified. If irreducible the neck may be opened
to reveal the contents and viability of the bowel inspected.

Warming of the bowel can lead to a decision if unsure of viability. (Ischaemic bowel should NOT be returned to the abdomen and should be resected with end-to-end anastomosis via a lower midline laparotomy.)

If unable to reduce the hernia then the lacunar ligament may be cut (watch for the obturator artery which sits behind).

The sac is then reduced and the neck transfixed using Vicryl suture, repair of the hernia opening is performed with nylon sutures between the medial inguinal and pectineal ligaments (take care to avoid the femoral vein laterally).

Closure The wound is closed in layers.

8 What are the specific complications of surgery?

- Immediate
  - Bowel ischaemia if there is reduction en masse or rough handling of the bowel
  - Damage to femoral vein
- Early
  - Infection
- Late
  - Recurrence

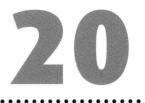

20

Haemorrhoidectomy

1 What are haemorrhoids and where do they occur?

They are caused by the engorgement of the internal haemorrhoidal venous plexus, which normally forms part of the anal cushions and may be internal (above the dentate line) or external (below the dentate line). They are normally found at 3, 7 and 11 o'clock in the lithotomy position.

2 What symptoms may be present?

Painless bleeding, discharge and irritation are common but large haemorrhoids may thrombose and infarct causing severe pain.

3 How are haemorrhoids classified?

1st degree	These bleed but do not prolapse
2nd degree	Prolapse on straining but reduce spontaneously
3rd degree	Prolapse on straining and only reduce with manual assistance
4th degree	Prolapsed and irreducible and may strangulate

4 Why should haemorrhoids be investigated?

Serious bowel pathology, for example a carcinoma or inflammatory bowel disease, must be excluded. Rectal examination, proctoscopy and sigmoidoscopy should therefore be performed in all cases.

5 What is the initial management of haemorrhoids?

Conservative treatments such as:

- Dietary advise (with increased fibre)
- Topical applicants
- Reduction of stool straining
- Laxatives if constipated

6 What treatment modalities are available in the outpatients department?

For 1st and 2nd degree haemorrhoids the following can be used:

- *Injection sclerotherapy*: About 2–3 ml of sclerosant (usually phenol in oil) is injected into the submucosal pedicle causing elevation of the submucosa and tissue necrosis.
- *Rubber band ligation*: During proctoscopy the haemorrhoid is identified and grasped using forceps. A band is applied at the base to strangulate the pile. This later sloughs off (this can also be used in 3rd degree haemorrhoids).

All of these procedures should be painless as they are performed above the dentate line.

7 When is a haemorrhoidectomy required?

This is usually indicated in severe cases that have been resilient to other treatments (<10%) such as large 3rd and 4th degree piles. Emergency operation can also be used to treat acute thrombosed and strangulated haemorrhoids to relieve the pain. There is a higher complication rate in this acute setting.

8 How do you perform a haemorrhoidectomy?

Position Lithotomy.

Procedure There are two techniques performed via anal retractors:

1 *Milligan Morgan*: The haemorrhoids are identified and dissected from the anal sphincter. The vascular pedicle is ligated and the wounds left open to granulate between bridges of skin and mucosa.
2 *Stapled haemorrhoidectomy*: A circular stapling gun is used to excise a doughnut of mucosa from the upper anal canal and lift the haemorrhoidal cushions back within the canal. It avoids a cutaneous incision and has a shorter operative time and recovery. It is best used for the smaller haemorrhoids but may have an increased complication rate.

Post-operatively Laxatives and a Metronidazole/GTN ointment should be given as well as suitable analgesia.

9 What are the complications specific to a haemorrhoidectomy?

- Immediate
  - Primary bleeding
  - Urinary retention
- Early
  - Pain
  - Infection

- Secondary bleeding (usually at 1 week when the clot falls away)
- Late
  - Anal stenosis
  - Incontinence

21

· · · · · · · · · · · · · · · · ·

Hip surgery

1 What options do you know for the management of OA of the hip?

- Conservative measures
  - Weight loss
  - Orthotics (walking sticks, shoe raises, etc.)
  - Physiotherapy
  - Occupational therapy
  - Lifestyle modifications
  - Analgesia or intra-articular corticosteroids
- Surgical measures
  - Total hip replacement (cemented, uncemented or hybrid)
  - Hip re-surfacing
  - Less commonly arthrodesis or osteotomies

2 Name three common approaches to the hip joint

These are described in relation to the gluteus medius muscle and are:

1 Lateral or the "Hardinge" approach (through the gluteus medius muscle)
2 Posterior approach
3 Anterior or the "Smith–Peterson" approach.

3 What layers does the surgeon travel through before reaching the hip joint in each of the above approaches?

Lateral	Posterior	Anterior
Skin	Skin	Skin
Subcutaneous fat	Subcutaneous fat	Subcutaneous fat
Fascia lata	Fascia lata	Fascia lata
	Trochanteric bursa	
Trochanteric bursa	Gluteus maximus	Plane between sartorius and TFL
Gluteus medius	Short ext. rotators	Capsule
Gluteus minimus	Capsule	
Capsule		

4 How do you approach the hip via the Hardinge approach?

Pre-operatively Consent is obtained appropriately, the side is marked and intravenous antibiotics are given at induction and for the first 24 hours post-operatively.

Position This is in the lateral position with the affected side on top. The surgeon stands behind the patient. The patient is secured in position with lumbar and pubic support as well as supports for the arms. Particular attention must be paid to prevent pressure necrosis and gel pads or wool must be placed in between tight fitting supports and bony prominences.

Incision The incision is made a hands breadth above and below the greater trochanter in line with the femur and with a slight proximal curve.

Approach This is as for the lateral approach (as discussed in Question 3) gluteus minimus and medius are detached from the greater trochanter and retracted anteriorly. The incision is extended proximally into the medius, which is split along the direction of its fibres and distally into vastus lateralis. Care is taken to avoid damage to the superior gluteal neurovascular bundle. The capsule is then fully exposed and incised to reveal the hip joint.

Closure This is in layers. It is important to achieve a good repair of the abductor tendons in an attempt to preserve hip abduction power. A drain may be placed in situ.

5 Describe the steps taken to expose the hip through the posterior approach

Pro-operative preparation, *position* and *closure* are as for the lateral approach.

Approach The skin and fascia are incised. The gluteus maximus and the short rotators (piriformis, gemelli, obturator externus and quadratus femoris) are identified and are detached from the greater trochanter. It is important to identify the sciatic nerve and protect it under the reflected short rotator muscles. The posterior capsule is then incised to expose the hip.

6 Discuss the advantages and the disadvantages of the Hardinge approach

The Hardinge approach is a simple approach with a good exposure of the hip joint for most hip operations. This makes judging the degree of anteversion of the femoral neck easy. It avoids close surgical dissection around the sciatic nerve and thus reduces the risk of damage to this nerve. This approach is said to have a lower incidence of post-operative dislocations as compared to the posterior approach.

The main criticism of this approach is the high likelihood of a Trendelenburg gait following surgery. This is mainly due to the fact that the abductors are detached during the approach but also the possibility of damage to the superior gluteal nerve.

7 What are the specific complications of a total hip replacement?

- Immediate
  - Haemorrhage
  - Intra-operative femoral fractures
  - Sciatic and gluteal nerve injury
- Early
  - Thrombosis
  - Wound infection
- Late
  - Deep infection
  - Dislocations
  - Wear of the implant
  - Aseptic loosening of the implant
  - Peri-prosthetic fractures

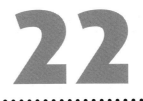

Hydrocele repair

1 What are hydroceles? What causes of hydroceles do you know?

A hydrocele is a collection of serous fluid in the tunica vaginalis. This can be due to:

- Decrease absorption of the fluid due to damage to scrotal venous or lymphatic systems following groin or scrotal surgery
- Increased production due to leaky vessels secondary to a malignant or inflammatory process
- A patent processus vaginalis
- Trauma

2 What pre-operative measures must be taken?

It is important to identify any underlying testicular pathology, in particular a testicular tumour. This is done by meticulous history taking and physical examination. The testicle is generally behind the hydrocele and can be palpated through the hydrocele. Further investigation by way of an ultrasound scan can be diagnostic.

3 What are the options in the management of a hydrocele?

- *Conservative*: This is to simply reassure the patient and may be an option if the hydrocele is asymptomatic, longstanding and after excluding any underlying pathology.
- *Aspiration*: This is a quick and easy option that can be performed in the clinic but has a high incidence of recurrence.
- *Surgical excision*: which can be either an extrusion procedure leaving the sac behind or using diathermy to excise the entire sac.

4 Name two surgical procedures used to repair a hydrocele? What is the main difference between the two?

Lord's and Jaboulay's procedures. In Jaboulay's the hydrocele sac is excised using diathermy and is associated with a greater degree of haematoma formation.

5 What layers are traversed when approaching the testes through the scrotum?

Skin
Subcutaneous fat
Dartos muscle
Colles fascia
External spermatic fascia
Cremasteric fascia
Internal spermatic fascia
Tunica vaginalis
Testis

6 Describe the Lord's procedure

Position The patient is placed supine on the operating table and routine preparation and draping of the groin is performed.

Incision A transverse incision is made across the hemiscrotum and the layers described in Question 5 are traversed. The fluid will then exit under pressure as the parietal layer of the tunica vaginalis is incised.

Procedure All the hydrocele fluid is suctioned out. Interrupted sutures are placed around the testis and the hydrocele sac is plicated. This is done by commencing each suture at the edge of the sac, picking up multiple layers of the sac before taking a bite of the tunica vaginalis close to the testis. This is repeated around the sac.

Closure After haemostasis is ensured. Closure is performed in layers, paying particular attention to the dartos layer. Topical antibiotic ointments can be applied to the wound.

7 What specific complications of this procedure do you know?

- Haematoma formation is common (large amounts can collect in the scrotum). There may be problems with cosmesis. The haematoma can also get infected.
- Wound infection.
- Recurrence.

23

The open repair of an inguinal hernia

1 How would you distinguish a direct from an indirect inguinal hernia?

- *Anatomically*: A direct inguinal hernia protrudes through the posterior wall of the inguinal canal medial to the inferior epigastric artery, whereas an indirect hernia emerges from the deep inguinal ring lateral to it.
- *Clinically*: An indirect inguinal hernia may be controlled by applying pressure on the abdominal wall at the site of the deep inguinal ring – surface marking: 1.5 cm above the mid-point of the inguinal ligament (midpoint of a line drawn from the pubic tubercle to the anterior superior iliac spine).

  Note: Not the midinguinal point (see Chapter 18, Femoral embolectomy).

2 What is the difference between an obstructed and a strangulated hernia?

An obstructed hernia contains obstructed but viable bowel, whereas a strangulated hernia may contain non-viable bowel since its venous drainage is compromised.

3 What pre-operative measures should be taken before the repair of an inguinal hernia?

- Consider general versus local anaesthetic. The procedure under a local anaesthetic is generally not advised in the anxious patient and in the obese patient. It is contraindicated in suspected strangulated herniae (where a more extensive dissection may be required).
- Consider an open versus laparoscopic repair. Laparoscopic repairs are generally chosen for bilateral or recurrent herniae.
- Two units of blood should be cross-matched and peri-operative intravenous antibiotics (e.g. Cefotaxime and Metronidazole) should be given in cases of strangulated herniae.
- The correct side should be marked.

4 How would you perform the open repair of an inguinal hernia?

Position This is supine. The patient is prepared and draped from his xiphoid process to the midthigh region.

Incision A groin incision is performed approximately 3 cm above and parallel to the medial two-thirds of the inguinal ligament.

The layers traversed are:

Skin
Subcutaneous fat
Scarpa's fascia
External oblique (dividing of which opens the inguinal canal)

Procedure The spermatic cord is located within the canal and separated from the hernial sac (thus carefully preserving the vas deferens). The sac is opened in indirect hernias (or directly reduced in direct) its contents inspected and reduced, and then transfixed at the deep ring.

- *The Bassini repair:* This approximates the conjoint tendon to the inguinal ligament from the pubic tubercle to the deep ring.
- *The Liechtenstein repair:* A prosthetic mesh (e.g. polytetrafluoroethane, PTFE) is sutured from the pubic tubercle to the inguinal ligament and the conjoint tendon, splitting to enclose the spermatic cord (a tension-free repair). This is the commonest method of repair.
- *The Shouldice repair:* A modification of the Bassini repair using a four-layer closure thereby doubling the transversalis fascia.

Closure The anterior abdominal wall is then closed in layers.

87

5 What are the specific complications associated with the repair of an inguinal hernia?

- Immediate
  - Haemorrhage
  - Injury to the ilioinguinal nerve
- Early
  - Wound infection
  - Ischaemic orchitis
- Late
  - Recurrence

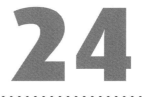

Laparotomy and abdominal incisions

1 On the sketch of the abdomen below label some of the common abdominal incisions and list their common indication.

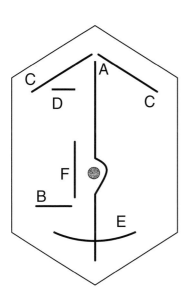

- **A:** Midline laparotomy used for access to the peritoneum. Upper or lower midline laparotomy incisions refer to the same incision only above or below the umbilicus, respectively.

- **B**: Lanz incision used in appendicectomy.
- **C**: Subcostal (Kocher's) incision used on the right for open cholecystectomy and on the left for a splenectomy.
- **D**: Right upper quadrant transverse incision also used for cholecystectomy.
- **E**: Pfannensteil incision used for access to pelvic viscera in gynaecology and urology.
- **F**: Paramedian incision

2 How do you perform a diagnostic laparotomy?

Pre-operatively General anaesthetic.

Position This is supine and the patient is prepared from the nipples to the groin.

Incision The layers traversed are:

Skin
Subcutaneous fat
Linea alba (thicker above umbilicus)
Fascia transversalis
Pre-peritoneal fat
Peritoneum

Procedure and inspection of abdomen The contents of the abdomen are inspected carefully and methodically beginning with the liver and spleen and then gently examining the stomach, the small bowel, and then the large bowel down to the rectum. Any abnormalities should be dealt with accordingly. If all is well then a final inspection of the pelvis is undertaken.

Closure The abdomen is closed with a mass closure technique (Jenkins rule) using, for example' a one-loop polydiaxone (PDS) suture and incorporating all of the above layers apart from the skin and superficial fat.

3 What is "Jenkins' rule"?

"Jenkins rule" describes the requirement of suture bites 1 cm in thickness and 1 cm apart. It is normal to require a length of suture 4× the length of the wound and it is also important to have the correct suture tension during closure to prevent wound dehiscence.

4 Describe a Kocher's incision

This is 2.5 cm below and parallel to the right costal margin.

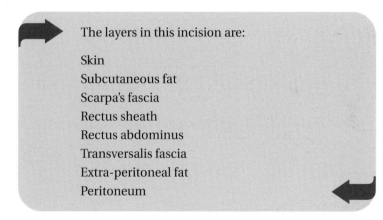

The layers in this incision are:

Skin
Subcutaneous fat
Scarpa's fascia
Rectus sheath
Rectus abdominus
Transversalis fascia
Extra-peritoneal fat
Peritoneum

5 What are the important complications specific to a laparotomy?

These also depend upon what procedure is required.
• Immediate
  • Haemorrhage

- Early
  - Peritonitis
  - Dehiscence of wound (technical failure)
- Late
  - Adhesions
  - Incisional hernia

Oesophago-gastro-duodenoscopy

1 Describe the important anatomical narrowings of the oesophagus

The oesophagus is a muscular tube approximately 25 cm long from the pharynx to the stomach. There are four anatomical narrowings to the oesophagus, these are listed proximal to distally. They may be visualised on oesophago-gastro-duodenoscopy (OGD) and are also the regions where foreign bodies may lodge and perforation are most likely to occur:

- Cricopharyngeal muscle
- Aortic arch
- Left main bronchus
- Lower oesophageal sphincter

2 What is an OGD and what are the advantages compared to contrast imaging?

OGD is the passage through the upper gastrointestinal (GI) tract using a flexible steerable fibre-optic telescope, which allows for direct visualisation of the tissues. The advantage over radiology is that a direct visualisation is achieved, early malignancies are detected (biopsy), exact identification of bleeding ulcers is achieved and therapy may be instituted.

3 What other therapies may be achieved during an OGD?

- Treatment of oesophageal strictures with dilatation techniques. The endoscope is passed into the oesophagus, the stricture is visualised and a wire passed through the stricture. The endoscope is then removed and increasing sized plastic dilators passed over the wire through the stricture until satisfactory clearance is achieved.
- Duodenoscopy allows for treatment of biliary tract disease.
- Percutaneous endoscopic gastrostomy (PEG) tube insertion.

4 Describe the steps undertaken in performing an OGD for a bleeding peptic ulcer

It must be first decided if the bleed is a low risk or high risk (e.g. Rockwall scoring system). If high-risk then an urgent OGD must be performed, if low-risk group the OGD should be done within 24 hours. The following must be considered:

- Adequate resuscitation with fluid and blood via $2\times$ large-bore cannulae
- Central venous catheter to estimate filling pressures and urinary catheter to measure output
- Blood transfusion
- Intravenous proton pump inhibitor
- Passage of the endoscope through the mouth and oesophagus to the stomach (transnasal route also available)
- Identification of the bleeding point
- Direct injection of adrenaline (1:10,000) $\pm$ sclerosants (this has however a 25% rebleed rate)

- If does the above does not work then laser or heat thermocoagulation
- If there is no haemostasis then definitive surgery should be performed

5 What are the specific complications to OGD?

- Sedation complications (especially elderly, liver disease, opioid treatment)
  - Oxygen, Naloxone and Flumazenil should be available
- Haemorrhage (on anticoagulants and biopsy taken)
  - Should be treated as stated above
- Perforation to pharynx, oesophagus, stomach and duodenum
  - High mortality rates if oesophageal perforation

The overall complication rate following OGD is low however at about 0.1%. It is a widely used diagnostic and therapeutic tool and tolerated well.

6 Describe ERCP (endoscopic retrograde cholangiopancreatography)

This entails using a duodenoscope with the aim of biliary tract cannulation and subsequent X-ray. It may be either diagnostic or therapeutic as mentioned below.

Pre-operatively The patient should be starved before the procedure

- Sedation given
- Local anaesthetic spray in throat
- IV antibiotics

Position This is in the left lateral position

Procedure The scope is passed into the duodenum and the ampulla is identified. A small cannula is inserted into the bile duct and pancreatic duct. Contrast solution (usually iodine) is then injected into the biliary tract with a subsequent radiograph taken. Possible therapies at this point are:

- Sphincterotomy and biliary stone extraction
- Stenting of malignant obstructions
- Stricture dilatation

7 What are the complications of ERCP?

- Perforation
- Haemorrhage
- Contrast reaction and anaphylaxis
- Infection and sepsis
- Pancreatitis

Orchidectomy

1 What two approaches do you know for performing an orchidectomy?

The two approaches for performing an orchidectomy are the scrotal or inguinal approaches.

2 Where do the lymphatics of the testis and the scrotal skin drain to respectively?

- The testis drains to the para-aortic lymph nodes at the level of L2.
- The scrotal skin drains via both the internal and external pudendal systems to the deep and superficial inguinal lymph nodes.

3 How does the above knowledge dictate the approach for orchidectomy for a testicular tumour?

As the scrotal skin and the testis have different blood supply and lymph drainage, an orchidectomy for a testicular tumour should be performed via an inguinal approach to avoid the possibility of tumour seeding to the deep and superficial inguinal systems.

4 What pre-operative measures must be taken prior to an orchidectomy?

- Informed consent (consider sperm banking)
- Clinical examination: tumour, other testis, hepatomegaly, lungs
- Tumour markers, liver and bone profile
- Chest X-ray (CXR)
- Scrotal ultrasound examining both testes
- Chest and abdominal CT scan (lungs, liver and para-aortic lymph nodes)
- Isotope bone scan

5 Briefly describe how you would perform an orchidectomy for testicular tumour

Position The patient is placed under a general anaesthetic and supine on the table. A routine preparation and draping of the groin is performed.

Incision and procedure A groin crease incision is made and is deepened into the inguinal canal by incising the external oblique aponeurosis (superficial inguinal ring). The spermatic cord is then identified and cross-clamped. It is important to clamp the cord prior to mobilising the testes to prevent squeezing tumour cells into the circulation. The cord is cut and the two ends ligated. The testis is then delivered through the inguinal canal by traction on the cord stump. The testis is released from its attachment to the scrotum and sent to histology.

Closure Haemostasis is ensured. Closure is in layers.

Note: A biopsy of the contralateral testis may also be performed.

6 What adjuvant treatment modalities can be undertaken?

- Radiotherapy: Seminomas are particularly sensitive and adjuvant radiotherapy after radical orchidectomy is standard management.
- Chemotherapy.
- Retroperitoneal lymph node surgery.

7 What other indications of orchidectomy do you know?

- Removal of a non-viable testis secondary to torsion, infection, etc.
- Bilateral orchidectomy as treatment for prostate cancer.

99

27

· · · · · · · · · · · · · · · · ·

Parotidectomy

1 What is the surface marking of the parotid gland?

The superior margin can be marked on the side of the face by a curved line starting at the tragus of the ear running to the middle of the cheek, just below the zygomatic arch. From here a curved line drawn down to the angle of mandible marks the anterior border. The inferior border is between the angle of the mandible and the mastoid process.

2 What different types of parotidectomy do you know? When are they performed?

A parotidectomy is performed to excise a tumour of the parotid gland. A *superficial parotidectomy* is undertaken either as a primary diagnostic procedure or as a curative procedure when only the superficial lobe is involved in small and low-grade tumours. In cases where the deep lobe is also involved and/or the tumour is known to be malignant a *conservative total parotidectomy* must be performed. This refers to the excision of the entire gland with conservation of the facial nerve. *Radical parotidectomy* with excision of the nerve is undertaken in cases of adherent or infiltrative disease.

3 What pre-operative considerations may be undertaken prior to a parotidectomy?

- Clinical assessment of the facial nerve to identify any pre-operative functional deficit
- Local examination and imaging to identify involved lymph nodes
- CT or MRI scanning to assess the deep lobe.
- Fine needle aspiration cytology (FNAC) to confirm the diagnosis
- CXR

4 How do you perform a parotidectomy?

Position The patient is placed supine with the head supported on a ring and tilted away from the affected side. Routine preparation is applied. It is important that draping leaves the face exposed to allow assessment of facial nerve function by visualising fascial muscle twitching.

Incision A pre-auricular incision is made (see diagram) curving behind the ear and to the mastoid process. From here the incision is curved again down the neck along the anterior border of the sternocleidomastoid muscle.

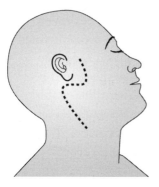

The layers travered are:

Skin
Subcutaneous fat
Platysma (in the distal part of the incision)
Parotid fascia or the investing layer of
deep cervical fascia
Parotid gland

Procedure Skin flaps are carefully elevated. It is important to identify and protect the facial nerve and its branches. The position of the nerve can be further ascertained by using a nerve stimulator. The superficial lobe is then dissected from the deep portion and excised. If the deep lobe is to be excised the facial nerve is carefully mobilised prior to its excision. The external carotid artery and/or the retromandibular vein may need to be ligated.

Closure The wound is closed in layers after absolute haemostasis is ensured and a suction drain is positioned.

5 List the anatomical features that help you identify the facial nerve in the above procedure

- Tragal or Conley's pointer, which is the cartilage of the external auditory meatus. The nerve lies about 1 cm medial and inferior to the tip of this pointer.
- Tympanomastoid suture that is easily palpable just in front of the mastoid process. The stylomastoid foramen (point of exit of the facial nerve) is just medial to this suture.
- The nerve bisects the angle created between the skull base and the posterior belly of the digastric muscle.

- Retrograde identification of the main trunk by first identifying the peripheral branches (temporal, zygomatic, buccal, mandibular or cervical).

6 What are the complications specific to a parotidectomy?

- Immediate
  - Facial nerve trauma, which can be a neuropraxia or more seriously permanent damage
  - Damage to the greater auricular nerve leading to numbness of the lower ear
  - Haemorrhage
- Early
  - Wound infection
- Late
  - Scarring
  - Frey's syndrome (this results in facial flushing or sweating during salivary stimulation and eating)

7 What is the anatomical basis of Frey's syndrome? How can it be treated?

This occurs due to the cross-regeneration of the damaged nerve fibres from the post-ganglionic secretomotor nerves of the parotid (parasympathetic) to the post-ganglionic fibres that supply the sweat glands (sympathetic).

The treatment involves reassurance and conservative measures in most instances, however local Botox injection or surgical division of the petrosal nerve (tympanic neurectomy) can be performed in severe cases.

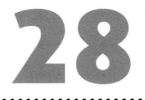

28

Perforated peptic ulcer

1 What are some of the common risk factors for peptic ulcer disease?

- *Helicobacter pylori* infection (in 90% of duodenal ulcer, DU)
- Alcohol abuse
- Non-steroidal anti-inflammatory drugs (NSAIDs)
- Steroids
- Old age

2 What pre-operative measures must be undertaken in the management of a patient with a perforated peptic ulcer?

- Intravenous fluid resuscitation
- Urinary catheterisation and hourly urine output monitoring
- Nasogastric intubation to decompress the stomach
- Central venous catheterisation (if the patient is haemo-dynamically unstable)
- Analgesia
- Intravenous proton pump inhibitors
- Intravenous antibiotics (e.g. Cefuroxime and Metronidazole)
- Blood investigations indicate a neutrophil leucocytosis (Pancreatitis must be excluded with an amylase)

- Erect CXR will reveal a pneumoperitoneum in only 80% of cases

  (Can also use a lateral decubitus film which is more sensitive)

3 Describe how you would repair a perforated DU

The aim is primarily to repair defect and to wash out the abdominal cavity.

Position This is supine the patient is prepared and draped as for a laparotomy.

Incision Upper midline through linea alba (see Chapter 24, Laparotomy).

Procedure The duodenum is isolated and the perforation identified. A patch of omentum is oversawn across the perforation using Vicryl sutures. The abdomen is irrigated with copious amounts of warm saline. A drain may be placed prior to closure.

Closure The abdomen is closed using mass closure technique as for a laparotomy.

4 What if there is a perforated gastric ulcer?

This will only be evident at operation and the treatment is the same as for DU. A biopsy of the ulcer should be taken for definitive pathological diagnosis prior to repair with an omental patch as there is a higher occurrence of malignant ulcer here.

Pyloric stenosis and Ramstedt's pyloromyotomy

1 What is idiopathic hypertrophic pyloric stenosis (IHPS)?

This is a congenital condition that presents in infants at around 6 weeks of age. There is hypertrophy of the circular muscle of the pylorus causing gastric outflow obstruction. It is a familial condition and seen especially in the first-born males. IHPS is considered a surgical emergency as the infant is unable to feed and loses large quantities of acidic gastric fluid leading to dehydration, alkalosis and electrolyte imbalances.

2 What is the biochemical abnormality in an infant with pyloric stenosis?

Hypochloraemic metabolic alkalosis. The serum potassium and sodium may also be decreased. There may even be a paradoxical acid urine as the kidneys excrete hydrogen ions in order to preserve potassium.

3 How is IHPS diagnosed?

Classically there is a history of non-bilious projectile vomiting, dehydration and failure to thrive. The child remains hungry after each vomiting. Clinically the thickened pylorus can be palpated in the epigastrium as an olive-sized mass. The diagnosis can be further supported with a test feed and confirmed on ultrasound scanning.

4 What is the management of an infant with pyloric stenosis?

- Fluid resuscitation using 0.45% normal saline with the addition of potassium chloride to each bag
- NGT insertion and regular aspiration of the gastric contents
- Surgery (Ramstedt's pyloromyotomy) after the alkalosis is corrected (typically after HCO_3 is below 25 mmol/l)

5 Describe the steps taken in performing a Ramstedt's pyloromyotomy

Position The infant is placed supine with whole abdomen prepared and draped.

Incision Usually a right upper quadrant cutting or muscle splitting incision is used (upper midline, umbilical and laparoscopic approaches may also be used). A small transverse incision is made 2 cm below the right costal margin.

> Layers traversed are:
>
> Skin
> Subcutaneous fat
> Fascia
> Rectus sheath/muscle
> Transversalis fascia
> Pre-peritoneal fat
> Peritoneum

Procedure The pyloric tumour is identified and the serosa dissected using either diathermy or a knife. The circular muscle is identified and split longitudinally taking care not to breach the underlying mucosa. The stomach is filled with air via the NGT to ensure that there has not been a mucosal breach. If this is found it should be repaired in a similar manner to duodenal perforations by using an omental patch.

Closure A mass abdominal closure is undertaken.

6 What are the complications specific to a pyloromyotomy?

- Immediate
  - Haemorrhage
  - Mucosal perforation
- Early
  - Infection
  - Persistent vomiting (occurs in 10% of cases and is usually self-limiting)
- Late
  - Incisional hernia

Right hemicolectomy

1 What pre-operative measures should be taken before a right hemicolectomy?

- Pre-operative investigations
  - To delineate the bowel anatomy (e.g. abdominal X-ray, barium enema, colonoscopy or a CT scan of the abdomen)
  - To assess the general condition of the patient (e.g. ECG, CXR, lung function tests or an echocardiogram)
- Group and save
- Consent
- Bowel preparation is not necessary
- Deep vein thrombosis (DVT) prophylaxis ("TEDS" stockings and peri-operative subcutaneous low-molecular-weight heparin)
- Peri-operative antibiotic prophylaxis

2 How do you perform a right hemicolectomy?

Position This is supine with the table tilted 20 degrees to the left, and the surgeon standing to the patient's left.

Incision The abdomen is draped and prepared as for a laparotomy and a midline laparotomy incision is made (see Chapter 24, Laparotomy).

Procedure After traversing the abdominal wall as for a laparotomy the peritoneum is entered and the colon is located. Clamps are placed on either side of the tumour to prevent intraluminal spread. The ascending colon is then mobilised by dividing the peritoneum, on its medial and lateral sides, up to the hepatic flexure. The following branches of the superior mesenteric artery are ligated and divided:

1 The ileocolic artery
2 The right colic artery
3 The right branch of the middle colic artery

A pair of "soft" clamps are then placed approximately 12 inches proximal to the ileocaecal valve and at the junction between the proximal and middle thirds of the transverse colon. A pair of "crushing" clamps are then placed 2 inches within the soft clamps and the bowel is divided and sent for histological examination. The ileum is then anastomised with the transverse colon (see Chapter 6, Principles of bowel anastomosis). Intraperitoneal lavage is carried out.

Closure The peritoneum and the anterior abdominal wall are closed as for a laparotomy (see Chapter 24, Laparotomy).

3 What major structures are at risk whilst performing a right hemicolectomy?

- The right gonadal artery and vein
- The right ureter and kidney
- The duodenum

4 What specific complications are associated with a right hemicolectomy?

- Immediate
  - Irresectable tumour

- Haemorrhage
- Damage to other structures (see Question 3 above)
- Early
  - Wound infection or peritonitis
  - Anastomotic leak
  - Bowel obstruction secondary to an anastomotic stricture or bowel ileus
- Late
  - Bowel obstruction secondary to adhesions
  - Tumour recurrence

31

. . . .

Skin cover (the reconstructive ladder)

1 List all the options available in providing cover to a skin wound

This is known as the reconstructive ladder starting with the simplest method and if not suitable moving on to the next (more complex) method aiming to achieve the best result.

1 Simple dressing and allowing healing by secondary intention
2 Direct primary closure
3 Delayed primary closure
4 Skin graft
5 Local flap
6 Free flap

2 What are the two main types of skin graft? What are the advantages and disadvantages of each?

The two main types are *full* or *partial* thickness skin graft.

Partial-thickness grafts are available in larger sizes and can be used to cover large defects, as the donor site does not require closure. They are also meshed which improves their ability to "take" and to conform to irregular shaped defects. In the long term however they have a poorer cosmetic outcome. There may also be problems with the donor site during the healing process.

Full-thickness grafts have a better cosmetic outcome and match the surrounding skin better. There are fewer problems with the donor site as they are closed directly. Full-thickness grafts are available in small sizes however and cannot be used to cover very large defects. For example the full-thickness grafts used to cover skin defects in the fingers, after a Dupuytrens dermatofasciectomy. These grafts are taken from the volar forearm skin.

3 What are the causes of skin graft failure and what measures are undertaken to counteract them?

- *Infection*   Presence of a high bacterial load can lead to graft failure. β-haemolytic streptococci are particularly linked to graft failure. If the bed is suspected to be infected grafting must be delayed whilst the infection is treated.

- *Sheering*   Friable small capillaries grow from the graft bed to supply the graft by around the 3rd day. Sheering and movement will lead to their disruption and graft failure. Grafts are therefore secured to the bed using peripheral sutures or clips. A secure dressing is also applied and left undisturbed for the first week.

- *Collections*   A haematoma or a seroma in between the graft and its bed can disrupt the blood supply leading to failure. Meticulous haemostasis prior to grafting, and meshing or slitting the graft to allow escape of any collection will therefore improve graft survival.

- *Graft bed*   This needs to be appropriate for grafting. Exposed tendons, bone and neuro-vascular structures can lead to graft failure. Alternative reconstructive methods may be required.

4 Give some examples of local flaps

- Simple advancement flaps
- Y–V advancement flaps
- Rotational flaps
- Transposition flaps

5 What do you understand by a free flap? Give an example

A free flap is a section of tissue that is taken from one part of the body together with its vascular pedicle and "grafted" to a defect in another part of the body. The vascular pedicle is anastomised to the host blood supply.

TRAM flap based on the inferior epigastric vascular pedicle used in breast reconstruction is one example of a free flap.

Spinal procedures

1 What are the common surgical approaches to the spine?

Posterior approaches These can be *midline* approaches over the spinous processes with retraction of the paraspinal muscles from the lamina using a cobb retractor. This gives good access to the posterior elements of the cervical, thoracic and lumbar spine. It is commonly used for lumbar discectomy, laminectomy and for posterior spinal instrumentation as it gives an easy route to the lamina and the pedicles.

A *costotransversctomy* approach provides a posterolateral approach to the thoracic spine through which the lateral aspect of the vertebral body and the anterior aspect of the spinal canal are reached without the need for a thoracotomy.

A *transpedicular* approach refers to creating a tunnel within the pedicle to allow access to the anterior elements.

A *paraspinal or wiltse* approach is a posterolateral approach to the lumbar spine that utilises the plane between the multifidus and longissimus muscles. This allows access to far lateral disc herniations without the need to resect joints.

Anterior approaches Anterior cervical approach, medial to sternocleidomastoid muscle, retracting the carotid sheath laterally and the trachea and the oesophagus medially, allows good access to the cervical spine as well as the T1 verteral body.

A thoracotomy (usually a left lateral thoracotomy) is used to access the T3–T12 vertebral bodies anteriorly. Anterior exposure of T2 and T3 vertebra is difficult, and options include a third-rid thoracotomy or a midline sterotomy.

A *transdiaphragmatic thoracolumbar approach* is used to access the anterior aspect of the thoracolumbar junction (T10–L2). The anterior aspect of the lumbar spine is accessed through abdominal incisions. This can be extra- or transperitoneal.

2 What are the indications for spinal surgery?

- *Decompression* of cord or nerve roots (disc herniation, spinal stenosis + collection, infection)
- *Stabilisation* if spinal integrity compromised (fractures, tumours)
- *Realignment* of spinal deformities (spondylolisthesis, scoliosis)

3 What conditions can be diagnosed by analysing the cerebrospinal fluid (CSF)?

- Infection
- Subarachnoid haemorrhage
- Central nervous system (CNS) malignancies
- Demyelinating disorders

4 At what spinal level should an lumbar puncture (LP) be performed? What is the surface marking of this level?

An LP can be performed at any level below the termination of the spinal cord (conus) this is usually the lower border of the first lumbar vertebrae. A common site for an LP however, is the space between the fourth and fifth lumbar vertebrae. The anatomical landmark for this point is the supracristal plane, which is a plane that transects the L4 spinous process and corresponds to the highest points of the iliac crests.

5 Describe how you would perform an LP

Position The patient can be placed in the lateral recumbent position or sat upright with the lower spine flexed. The skin is cleaned and the area prepared and draped.

Procedure An appropriate size spinal needle is used. The needle is entered in the midline and in the space between the L4 and L5 spinous processes (see above) with the needle directed caudally. The needle is advanced into the subarachnoid space and the position is confirmed with backflow of CSF.

The layers the needle traverses are:

Skin
Subcutaneous fat
Interspinous ligament
Ligamentum flavum
Epidural fat
Dura mater (gives a characteristic "pop" as enters here)
Subarachnoid space

It is usually about 4–6 cm from the skin to the dura in the average person.

A manometer is attached; the pressure is recorded and up to 40 ml of CSF may normally be withdrawn safely. This is sent for protein, glucose, microscopy and culture.

6 What are the complications of LP?

- Acute
  - Haemorrhage
  - Tonsillar herniation (if there is raised intracranial pressure in the posterior cranial fossa)
- Early
  - Radicular pain or numbness
  - Headache (seen in 30%. This can be minimised with 4-hour recumbancy post-LP)
  - CNS infection
- Late
  - Epidermoid formation

Splenectomy

1 List some of the common indications for a splenectomy

- Trauma (around 30% of cases)
- Hypersplenism: where blood products are destroyed within the spleen, for example:
  - Immune thrombocytopenic purpura (ITP)
  - Hereditary spherocytosis
  - Autoimmune haemolytic anaemia
- Neoplasia
  - Lymphoma (staging)
  - Leukaemia
  - Gastric or pancreatic tumours (splenectomy as part of radical surgery)
- Splenic cysts
- Splenic abscess

2 Which vaccination or antibiotic prophylaxis do you consider for a patient undergoing an elective splenectomy?

- *Vaccination*: "Triple vaccination" should be offered to all patients at least 2 weeks prior to surgery:
  - *Streptococcus pneumoniae* vaccine to all patients

- *Haemophilus influenzae* vaccination if not previously received
- *Meningococcal* vaccination.
- *Antibiotics*: Life-long antibiotic prophylaxis with phenoxy-penicillin should be offered to all patients. This is particularly important in the first 2 years following surgery. Erythromycin is given in cases of penicillin allergy.

3 Describe three important peritoneal attachments, knowledge of which is essential in performing a splenectomy

1 *Lieno-renal ligament*, which attaches the splenic hilum to the left kidney. It contains branches of the splenic artery within it.
2 *Gastro-splenic ligament*, which attaches the splenic hilum to the greater curvature of the stomach.
3 *Phrenico-colic ligament*, which forms the upper margin of the left paracolic gutter and connects the colon to the peritoneum on the left hemi diaphragm. The spleen also has attachments to this ligament.

4 How do you perform an open splenectomy?

Position This is supine with the surgeon on the right of the patient. The abdomen is prepared and draped as for a laparotomy. An NGT is inserted to empty the stomach.

Incision A midline or a left subcostal (Kocher) incision is made and deepened to enter the peritoneum (see Chapter 24, Laprotomy and abdominal incisions).

Procedure In trauma free blood is evacuated and a quick examination of the intra-abdominal organs is performed to identify any other source for bleeding. A hand is placed behind the spleen and the spleen is drawn medially. The attachments to the diaphragm are divided to facilitate this. The lieno-renal ligament is then ligated and divided. The spleen can now be mobilised and delivered into the incision. The splenic artery, vein and the short gastric vessels are ligated and divided. Care is taken to avoid injury to the tail of the pancreas. The spleen is then removed. Any spenules should be looked for and removed if the procedure is done for haematological reasons.

Closure This is in layers as described in abdominal incisions section. A drain may be used.

5 How do you perform a laparoscopic splenectomy?

Position This is with the patient in the lateral position secured with table supports.

Incision Four or five laparoscopic ports are made and an angled telescope is introduced through the umbilical port.

Procedure Lower pole vessels are ligated first before dissection is carried out in the hilum. The splenic vessels are clipped and divided. The short gastric vessels are then identified and divided after ligation with clips. Any remaining peritoneal attachments are divided before the spleen is removed. Retrieval is by placing the spleen in a bag and removing it through one of the larger port sites. Larger spleens may need to be fractured to aid retrieval.

Closure All of the port sites are closed in layers.

6 What are the complications of splenectomy?

- Haemorrhage
- Gastric dilatation (NGT post-operatively)

- Pancreatic fistula
- Subphrenic abscess/collection
- Rebound neutrophilia
- Thrombocytosis (increased risk of thrombosis)
- Overwhelming sepsis

7 What particular infections are post-splenectomy patients at risk of?

- Malaria
- Encapsulated organisms (e.g. *Streptococcus pneumoniae, Haemophilus influenzae, Neisseria meningitidis*)

126

Stomas

1 What is a stoma?

A stoma is a surgically created opening of bowel or urinary tract to an external surface.

2 What different types of stoma do you know?

- Loop colostomy or ileostomy.
- End colostomy or ileostomy.
- Urostomy – to divert urine used after a cystectomy to collect urine from the ureters.
- Gastrostomy or jejunostomy – used for feeding patients with functioning gut that are unable to take food orally.
- Caecostomy – that is created by intubating the caecum with a Foley catheter usually through the appendicular stump after performing an appendicectomy.

3 Where should the stoma be sited?

It is necessary to plan the exact site of stoma pre-operatively by involving the patient. This has been shown to improve outcome. The optimal site of stoma placement should be marked pre-operatively. This should be on flat skin, away from scars and avoiding bony prominences and the umbilicus. The positioning of the patients clothing should also be taken into account.

There is usually a stoma therapist on site for this.

4 Where are stomas normally sited?

The usual site is halfway between the umbilicus and the anterior superior iliac spine in the iliac fossa. Ileostomies are usually sited on the right and colostomies on the left.

5 In what circumstances are temporary stomas used?

Temporary loop stomas are used to allow diversion of faeculant material away from a distal part of the bowel to allow healing of an anastomosis or fistula. Common types include loop ileostomies following anterior resection.

Temporary end colostomies are used following a Hartmann's procedure and although deemed reversible, are only actually reversed in about 50% of cases.

6 What stoma is used in a Hartmann's procedure?

This is performed after resection of the sigmoid colon and when due to perforation and peritonitis, a primary anastomosis is contraindicated. The rectal stump is oversawn and an end colostomy is fashioned by using the descending colon. The rectal stump is either left in the abdomen or is brought out to the skin and fashioned as a mucous fistula.

7 Describe the formation of an ileostomy

Position Supine as for a laparotomy. The site is marked pre-operatively.

Incision After the primary procedure is performed (e.g. a panproctocolectomy) a 2–3-cm skin disc is removed in the right iliac fossa.

Procedure The incision is deepened through the rectus abdominus and down to the parietal peritoneum. This is then incised and the pre-clamped ileum is located and brought out of the abdomen. The main abdominal wound is closed. The ileal clamp is removed. The stoma is fashioned by suturing the serosa, seromuscular layer and the skin with Vicryl. This everts the ileal stump and creates a spout, which should be about 6 cm long in order to protect the skin from the irritant ileal fluid (see diagram).

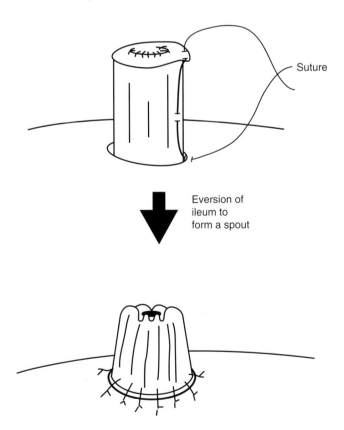

Suture

Eversion of
ileum to
form a spout

Closure An ileostomy bag is placed over the stoma and monitored for drainage.

8 What complications arise from stomas?

- Immediate
  - Bleeding
  - Ischaemia/necrosis: This is generally the result of technical failure and is usually if the stoma is formed under tension or a poor blood supply
- Early
  - High output: Ileostomies may put out more fluid than expected (normal 500ml/day) with massive salt and water loss, which must be corrected
  - Obstruction
  - Retraction (especially loop colostomy)
- Late
  - Obstruction
  - Prolapse
  - Parastomal herniation
  - Fistula formation (especially with ileostomies)
  - Skin irritation (especially with ileostomies)
  - Psychological

Submandibular gland excision

1 What are the borders of the submandibular triangle?

The submandibular triangle is a subsection of the anterior triangle of the neck formed by the digastric muscle. It contains the submandibular salivary gland.

The superior border is the inferior border of the mandible and is inferiorly bordered on the medial side by the anterior belly of digastric and on the lateral side by its posterior belly.

2 How do you perform an excision of the submandibular gland?

Position The patient is placed supine, the head supported and tilted away from the operative side. Routine skin preparation and draping is performed.

Incision An incision is made parallel and at least 2 cm below the inferior edge of the posterior half of the mandible.

Procedure The incision is deepened through:

> Skin
> Subcutaneous fat
> Platysma
> Investing layer of deep cervical fascia
> (gland capsule)

The deep fascia is reflected superiorly to expose the superficial lobe of the gland. The facial artery is ligated as it curves over the gland. To reach the deep part of the gland mylohyoid muscle is retracted. The submandibular salivary duct is identified and ligated taking care to preserve the lingual nerve, which lies close to it. The hypoglossal nerve can be seen lying deep to the gland on the surface of the hypoglossus muscle. The entire gland is then removed. The surrounding fat and soft tissue must also be excised to ensure adequate excision margins.

Closure The wound is closed in layers and a suction drain positioned.

3 Why must the skin incision be placed well below the inferior margin of the mandible?

The incision is placed here to avoid damaging the marginal mandibular branch of the facial nerve, which runs superficial to the investing layer of deep fascia and close to the inferior margin of the mandible.

4 What is the consequence of the division of the marginal mandibular branch of the facial nerve?

This nerve supplies the depressor anguli oris muscle that, as its name implies, acts to depress the corner of the mouth. Division of the nerve and subsequent paralysis of the muscle leads to an unopposed elevation of the angle of the mouth by the antagonistic levator anguli oris muscle.

5 What structures are at risk during submandibular gland excision?

- Marginal mandibular branch of facial nerve (if the skin incision is misplaced)
- Lingual nerve
- Hypoglossal nerve
- Nerve to mylohyoid

Tendon repairs

1 Why are repair of flexor tendons in the hand challenging?

This is because they are contained in well-lubricated synovial sheaths therefore:

- After lacerations they can readily retract a longer distance proximally.
- The repair must allow free gliding of the tendon within its sheath to ensure a normal function.
- Damage to the sheath and the various pulleys can result in bow stringing of the affected tendons reducing grip strength.
- Unsatisfactory post-repair rehabilitation may result in adhesions within the sheath resulting in inadequate function.

2 Describe the different zones of flexor tendon injuries in the hand

- *Zone I* Distal to the insertion of flexor digitorum superficialis (FDS) thus only contains the flexor digitorum profundus (FDP) tendon in the flexor sheath.
- *Zone II* This zone is from the beginning of the flexor sheath in the distal palm proximally to the start of Zone I

distally. Zone II contains both the FDP and FDS tendons in the flexor sheath.

- *Zone III* This zone starts distal to the carpal tunnel and end at the beginning of Zone II thus containing all the tendons free from synovial sheath in the palm.
- *Zone IV* This is the carpal tunnel with the tendons lying under the flexor retinaculum.
- *Zone V* This refers to the tendons proximal to the carpal tunnel in the forearm.

3 Describe a technique for repair of a tendon

A core suture (Kessler repair) is used, ensuring that the knot is within the tendon as illustrated. This will reduce the bulk of the repair and allow easier gliding of the tendon. This is augmented by smaller circumferential sutures.

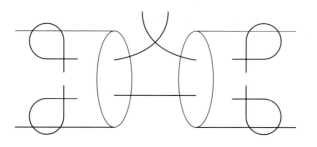

37

Thoracostomy (insertion of a chest drain)

1 What are the indications for insertion of a chest drain?

The main purpose of a chest drain is to remove or prevent the collection of pleural contents that result in ventilatory compromise. Some of the indications are listed below:
- Pneumothorax
- Haemothorax
- Pleural effusion (infective, malignant, congestive)
- Empyema
- Chest trauma (especially those with open or penetrating chest wounds)
- Chylothorax
- Post-operative (prophylactic)
- Prior to positive pressure ventilation

2 What surface makings help in deciding the site of chest drain insertion?

The safe site for a chest drain is within an imaginary triangle on the side of the chest wall, and, on the *superior border* of the rib that forms the inferior border of the chosen intercostal space.

The three sides of this triangle are marked anteriorly by the lateral border of the pectoralis major muscle, posteriorly by the *anterior axillary* line and inferiorly by the sixth rib.

3 What are the anatomical reasons for the site chosen in Question 2?

- Intercostal neurovascular bundles are at the *inferior border* of the rib and away from the site of tube insertion.
- The long thoracic nerve is marked by the *midaxillary* line and thus outside the above triangle.

4 Describe how you would insert an intercostal chest drain

Position The patient is placed supine at a 45-degree angle and tilted away from the side of the procedure. The shoulder is then abducted (resting hands on top of head) to allow better access to the chest wall. The area is prepared with antiseptic fluid, local anaesthesia infiltrated and draped in an aseptic manner.

Note that other positions are possible, for example patients can be asked to sit forward resting their arms on a table in front.

Incision A 2-cm incision is made in the appropriate position (discussed in Question 2) usually within the fourth or fifth intercostal spaces and deepened through:

Skin
Subcutaneous fat
Fascia
Serratus anterior
External intercostals
Internal intercostals
Innermost intercostals
Endothoracic fascia
Parietal pleura
Pleural space

139

Procedure The intercostal layers are dissected bluntly using a haemostat until the pleural space is reached. This is confirmed by the expulsion of a gush of air. A finger is then used to sweep the thoracic cavity ensuring the lung is away from the chest wall. The tube can now be passed through the track. It is safe practice to discard the trocar and use a sponge holder to insert the tube. The free end of the tube is then connected to a sealed underwater drainage system.

Closure A large non-absorbable suture is used to secure the tube to the skin before appropriate adhesive dressings are applied. A second suture is also placed in the form of a purse-string to aid closure at the time of drain removal. A CXR will confirm correct positioning.

5 List some of the specific complications of inserting a tube thoracostomy

- Bleeding
- Infection (superficial skin or empyema)
- Visceral perforation (heart, lungs, great vessels)
- Abdominal placement (which may lead to abdominal visceral perforation)
- Surgical emphysema
- Tube blockage (this can result in life-threatening tension pneumothorax)
- Pulmonary oedema (due to rapid re-expansion of a collapsed lung)

6 Describe how you would remove a chest drain

- Adherent dressings or tape is removed
- The entry site is cleaned using antiseptic fluid
- The suture securing the drain to the skin is cut avoiding damage to the purse-string suture
- The patient is asked to maintain a "deep breath in" to ensure maximal expansion of the lung and at the same time the drain is removed
- The purse-string suture is tied
- Adhesive dressings are applied

Thoracotomy

1 List some of the common approaches to the thoracic cavity. What are the common indications of each?

Approach	Common indication
Median sternotomy	CABG, other cardiac surgery, excision of thymoma
Posterolateral thoracotomy	Elective pulmonary surgery (lung resection)
Anterolateral thoracotomy	Trauma (on left gives rapid access to pericardium) also lobar resections or lung biopsy
Clamshell thoracotomy	Access to both pleural cavities (lung transplant)
Thoracoscopy	Lung biopsy, sympathetic neurectomy, pleurectomy

2 Describe the median sternotomy approach

Position The patient is placed supine with both arms on the side. The chest is shaved and prepared in the routine manner.

Incision A longitudinal incision is made starting from the sternal notch to two fingers breaths below the xiphoid process. The incision is deepened through to the sternum.

Procedure The sternum is marked using diathermy in its midline to aid an accurate midline sternotomy. The xiphoid process is cut longitudinally with heavy scissors before engaging a reciprocating saw to divide the sternum in its midline. Blunt dissection with a finger behind the sternum will aid engagement of the saw. Ventilation must be ceased during the sawing process to reduce the risk of pleural injury. A sternal retractor will then give a good exposure of the thoracic cavity. A fatty layer from the thymus remnant is divided before reaching the pericardium.

The layers traversed are therefore:

Skin
Subcutaneous fat
Midline fascia connecting the pectoralis major muscles on each side
Periosteum
Sternum
Thymic remnant
Pre-pericardial fat
Parietal pericardium

Closure The sternum is closed using interrupted steel wire sutures. The fascia, fat and skin are then closed in separate layers.

3 List the possible conduits used as coronary artery bypass grafts

- Long saphenous vein
- Left internal mammory artery (LIMA)

- Right internal mammory artery (RIMA)
- Radial artery
- Short saphenous vein
- Cephalic vein

4 Describe the posterolateral thoracotomy approach

Position The patient is placed in the lateral position and secured to the table with supports. A double lumen endotracheal tube is used to for lung surgery. Routine preparation and draping is performed.

Incision An incision is made over the fourth or fifth intercostal space starting at a point about one finger breath medial to the medial border of the scapula to a point 2 cm below the scapula tip and curved to the midaxillary line and deepened through fat and fascia.

Procedure The latissimus dorsi muscle is then exposed and divided in the line of the incision. This exposes the serratus anterior muscle anteriorly and a fatty layer posteriorly which are again incised to expose the underlying ribs and intercostal muscles. Serratus anterior is left intact and retracted only, in the popular "muscle-sparing" approach. The intercostal muscle is divided using diathermy on the top of the lower rib of the chosen intercostal space and the pleural cavity entered.

> The layers traversed are therefore:
>
> Skin
> Subcutaneous fat
> Pectoral fascia
> Latissimus dorsi muscle
> Serratus anterior muscle
> External intercostal muscle
> Internal intercostal muscle
> Parietal pleura
> Visceral pleura
> Lung

Closure The ribs are approximated using heavy sutures that are passed around them and tied. The serratus anterior and latissimus dorsi muscles are repaired before the subcutaneous tissues and skin are closed in layers.

144

5 What is an emergency thoracotomy and when should it be performed?

This is a thoracotomy that is performed in the emergency room, as the patient is too unstable for transfer to the operating theatre. A number of different approaches may be used. An emergency thoracotomy is indicated in a patient with:

- Penetrating chest injury resulting in cardiac tamponade
- Massive, abdominal haemorrhage for aortic cross-clamping
- Massive, uncontrollable haemorrhage into airways from intrathoracic vessels

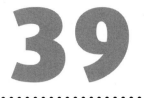

Thyroidectomy

1 What is the arterial and venous supply to the thyroid gland?

Arterial supply Superior and inferior thyroid arteries on both sides. The superior thyroid artery is a branch of the external carotid and the inferior thyroid artery is a branch of the thyro-cervical trunk, which in turn is a branch of the subclavian artery. At times the single thyroid ima artery, which is a direct branch of the brachiocephalic trunk, may be present in the midline.

Venous supply This is via the superior, middle and inferior thyroid veins on both sides. The former two drain into the internal jugular veins whereas the inferior thyroid veins drain into the brachiocephalic veins.

2 What specific pre-operative measures are taken prior to a thyroidectomy for thyrotoxicosis?

- Patients must be made euthyroid
- Vocal cord assessment using indirect laryngoscopy
- Biochemical analysis of calcium metabolism pre-operatively
- β-blockers may also be considered in an unstable patient
- In large retro-sternal goitres a CT scan is performed to assess tracheal deviation and the extent of retro-sternal extension

- Iodine for 2 weeks pre-operatively can reduce the vascularity of the gland

3 What different types of thyroidectomy do you know?

- Hemithyroidectomy (lobectomy or isthmusectomy)
- Total thyroidectomy (subtotal, near total or total)

4 What is a subtotal thyroidectomy?

Subtotal thyroidectomy refers to the excision of the entire gland but leaving about 4 g of thyroid tissue on each side. It is thought that this will reduce the risk of damage to the recurrent laryngeal nerves as well as protecting the parathyroids. There is also enough thyroid tissue left behind to avoid post-operative thyroid hormone replacement.

5 How does one perform a thyroidectomy?

Position Is supine with the neck extended and the head supported on a ring. The table is tilted 20–30 degrees "head up" to aid in emptying the neck veins. Routine skin preparation and draping is performed.

Incision A transverse incision is made in a skin crease at a point midway between the suprasternal notch and the thyroid cartilage.

> The following layers are traversed:
>
> Skin
> Subcutaneous fat
> Platysma
> Investing layer of cervical fascia (divided longitudinally, in the midline)
> The midline fascia connecting the strap muscles on each side
> Pre-tracheal fascia
> Thyroid

The skin flaps are elevated and retracted using a Joll's retractor. The strap muscles (sternothyroid and the deeper sternothyroid) are elevated and retracted for maximum exposure of the gland.

Procedure The middle thyroid vein is ligated and divided. The superior thyroid vein and artery are identified and ligated protecting the external laryngeal nerve. The inferior thyroid artery (and vein) are then identified and ligated close to the gland avoiding the recurrent laryngeal nerve and after careful identification of the parathyroid glands. The thyroid gland is then mobilised and removed.

Closure Careful haemostasis is paramount. A suction wound drain can be used. The strap muscles and the platysma are approximated with absorbable sutures and the skin is closed.

6 What are the specific complications of this procedure?

- Most common nerve injury is damage to the external branch of superior laryngeal nerve leading to a subtle disturbance in voice and in particular singing

- Damage to the recurrent laryngeal nerve (see below)
- Haemorrhage which can lead to life-threatening airway compromise
- Hypocalcaemia due to inadvertent damage to the parathyroids
- Hypothyroidism requiring thyroid hormone replacement
- Thyroid storm

7 What does the recurrent laryngeal nerve supply and what is the consequence of its division?

The recurrent laryngeal nerve provides the motor supply to the vocal cords (all intrinsic muscles of the larynx with the exception of cricothyroid) and sensory supply to the mucous membrane of the larynx inferior to the vocal folds.

Unilateral division will result in noticeable voice changes and reduced coughing ability. Bilateral division will result in both cords adopting an adducted position that can lead to upper airway obstruction post-operatively.

40

. . . .

Tracheostomy

1 When may a tracheostomy be indicated?

A tracheostomy may be indicated in a patient when:

- The upper airway is compromised due to:
  - Trauma: maxillofacial fractures, major ENT surgery
  - Infection: epiglottitis
  - Tumour: laryngeal cancer
  - Inflammation: angioedema
  - Neurological: bilateral recurrent laryngeal nerve palsy
  - Congenital: subglottic stenosis
- Long periods of endotracheal intubation is expected
- He/she cannot tolerate intubation without sedation
- Severe respiratory disease (e.g. chronic obstructive airways disease, COAD) is present, to reduce the work of breathing by reducing anatomical dead space.

2 What different types of tracheostomy do you know?

- Open surgical tracheostomy
- Percutaneous tracheostomy
- Translaryngeal tracheostomy

3 How would you perform an open surgical tracheostomy?

Position General or local anaesthesia can be used. The patient is placed supine on the operating table with the neck in slight extension. The operative field is prepared and draped in the routine manner.

Incision A transverse skin crease incision is made midway between the suprasternal notch and the cricoid cartilage and deepened through:

> Skin
> Subcutaneous fat
> Platysma
> Investing layer of deep cervical fascia
> Midline fascia connecting the strap muscles (incised longitudinally)
> Pre-tracheal fascia
> Thyroid isthmus
> Trachea

Procedure The strap muscles are retracted laterally to expose the thyroid isthmus, which is transfixed and divided. The cricoid and the first tracheal ring should not be damaged to prevent subglottic stenosis in the future. A Björk flap (distally based tracheal flap) is made by excising the 2nd, 3rd and 4th tracheal rings. A cuffed tracheostomy tube is then placed within the tracheal lumen.

Closure The tube is sutured to skin and secured. The cuff is inflated and the skin wound closed loosely around the tube. The tube should also be secured using tapes around the neck.

In an emergency setting a longitudinal midline incision provides rapid access and may be preferred to the transverse approach described above.

4 What is percutaneous tracheostomy?

This is a technique used by the critical care physicians. It involves placing a cannula into the trachea at the level of the 2nd or 3rd ring. A guidewire is then inserted through the cannula and the cannula is removed. The puncture site is then dilated using dilating instruments until it is large enough to accept a tracheostomy tube. Simultaneous fibre-optic visualisation may be used to ensure correct positioning.

5 What are the pros and cons of the technique described in Question 4?

This is a quick procedure that does not require the presence of a surgeon and can be performed on the ICU. It is safer in patients with coagulopathy and has been said to have fewer post-operative complications such as subglottic stenosis. It is also cosmetically more acceptable.

On the other hand, percutaneous tracheostomy is a relatively new technique. Correct placement needs to be confirmed by fibre-optic bronchoscopy and if a complication does occur the presence of the surgeon is still required.

6 What are the complications of a tracheostomy?

- Immediate
  - Haemorrhage
  - Air embolism

- Damage to adjacent structures:
  - Dome of pleura (especially in children)
  - Recurrent laryngeal nerves
  - Brachiocephalic vein
- Early
  - Wound infection
  - Surgical emphysema
  - Pneumonia
  - Blockage or displacement of tube
- Late
  - Tracheal or subglottic stenosis
  - Fistulas
  - Keloid or hypertrophic scars

7 What different types of tracheostomy tubes are there?

- Cuffed or uncuffed
- Fenestrated or non-fenestrated: fenestrations allow passage of air over the vocal cords and will therefore allow phonation and speech.

41

· · · · · · · · · · · · · · · ·

Urinary retention and related surgical procedures

1 What different types of urinary catheters do you know?

- Latex catheters
- Silicone catheters (more suitable for long-term use)
- Three-way catheters used for irrigation of the bladder
- In/out catheters (single lumen) used for intermittent self-catheterisation (ISC)
- Beaked Coude catheter

2 How would you insert a male urethral catheter?

Position After explaining the procedure and obtaining consent the patient is placed supine and the genitals are cleaned using antiseptic solution. The foreskin must be retracted to clean the glans. Sterile drapes are used to cover the groin.

Procedure Local anaesthetic gel is inserted into the urethra through its meatal opening. The urethra should be held closed with firm pressure to allow the anaesthetic to take effect. The catheter is then inserted into the urethra and through the prostate and advanced as far as possible to ensure the bladder is reached. Once in the bladder urine will start to drain. A suitable catheter bag is connected to the catheter. The balloon is then inflated using an appropriate volume (10 ml if using an ordinary Foley catheter) of water.

Closure The patient is cleaned and the bag secured. A urinary sample is sent for microscopy and the residual volume of urine is noted and documented. Remember to pull back the foreskin to avoid the development of a paraphimosis.

3 How do you insert a suprapubic catheter?

Position After explaining the procedure and obtaining consent the patient is placed supine. It is important to examine the abdomen to ensure distension of the bladder. The lower abdomen is cleaned with an antiseptic solution and the area draped.

Procedure A suitable volume of local anaesthetic (e.g. 10 ml of 2% lidocaine) is infiltrated. The infiltration is made in the midline below the umbilicus and a point two to three fingers breaths above the pubic symphysis. It is good practice to advance the needle deep, infiltrating the deeper layers as well as aspirating urine from the bladder to ensure correct placement of the catheter. A 2-cm transverse incision is made through the skin. A trocar is then inserted into the bladder with firm but controlled pressure. The trocar is removed but the plastic track is retained and the catheter inserted through this track. The catheter balloon is then inflated by injecting an appropriate volume of water.

Closure A catheter bag is connected. The plastic track is removed and the catheter is secured to the skin with non-absorbable sutures.

4 What is the relationship of the peritoneum to the urinary bladder and how is this utilised when inserting a suprapubic catheter?

In both male and female the bladder is the most anterior pelvic viscus. The peritoneum covers its dome and part of its posterior wall. Anteriorly the peritoneum reflects up against the anterior abdominal wall leaving the anterior wall of the bladder extraperitoneal. The distended bladder rises into the abdomen and in doing so brings its anterior wall in direct contact with the anterior abdominal wall. A suprapubic catheter can therefore be safely inserted without breaching the peritoneum.

5 What surgical approaches are used for the resection of the prostate?

155

- TURP (Transurethral resection of prostate)
- Retropubic prostatectomy (used with very large glands (>100 g) or with radical surgery for malignancy)

6 What are the complications of TURP?

- Haemorrhage, which can be immediate, primary or secondary. Secondary haemorrhage occurs typically around the tenth post-operative day and is self-limiting. Early bleeding may lead to clot retention and bladder irrigation is of outmost importance.
- Retrograde ejaculation may occur in up to 75% of patients. This is not a problem in the elderly or in patients who have completed their family but can cause anxiety and patients should therefore be appropriately informed pre-operatively.
- Infection.
- Impotence.

- Incontinence.
- TURP syndrome.

7 What is TURP syndrome and how is it prevented?

This refers to the systemic absorption of the irrigation fluid during TURP and leads to hypervoleamia, hypertension, hyponatraemia and eventually cerebral oedema, confusion and death. To prevent it the duration of surgery must be limited and measures under taken to reduce the intravesical pressure. One such measure is to reduce the height of the irrigation bags to below 1 m. Modern fluids are isotonic glycine and are kept warm to prevent haemolysis and hypothermia, respectively.

8 What are the limits of resection in a TURP and why?

The resection must not go beyond:

- The verumontanum (prominent portion of the male urethra on which lies the opening of the prostatic utricle and, on either side of it, the orifices of the ejaculatory ducts) distally as this results in retrograde ejaculation.
- The pink transverse fibres of the prostatic capsule as capsular perforation increase the risk of TURP syndrome.

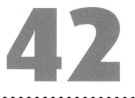

Varicose vein surgery

1 What is the aetiology of varicose veins?

The aetiology of varicose veins can be primary (95%) or
secondary:

- Primary varicose veins are caused by incompetence of valves
  in the connecting veins between the deep and superficial
  venous systems. This leads to back flow of blood from the
  deep into the superficial veins leading to an increase in pressure and development of varicosities.
- Secondary varicose veins develop due to occlusion of the
  deep system (thrombosis) leading to diversion of venous flow
  to the superficial veins.

2 What are the common sites of venous incompetence?

- Sapheno-femoral junction between the greater saphenous
  vein and the femoral vein in the groin (90%)
- Sapheno-popliteal junction between the greater saphenous
  vein and the popliteal vein in the popliteal fossa
- Midthigh perforator
- 2–3 perforators in the calf

3 What is the surface marking of the greater saphenous vein?

The greater or long saphenous vein (LSV) starts at the midportion of the medial arch of the foot. It ascends anterior to the medial malleolus on the medial aspect of the lower leg. At the knee it passes about a hand's breath behind the medial femoral condyle before passing towards the anteromedial thigh. It joins the femoral vein at the sapheno-femoral junction medial to the femoral artery (femoral pulse) about 3 cm below the inguinal ligament.

4 List some of the specific pre-operative measures that should be undertaken prior to surgery

- Ensure that the deep venous system is patent by performing a duplex ultrasound. Removing the superficial veins in a patient with non-functioning deep veins can lead to devastating venous hypertension.
- Identify and mark the location of the incompetent perforating veins (Trendelenburg test, duplex or Doppler).
- Mark all of the varicosities prior to anaesthesia and with the patient standing.

5 Describe the steps taken in performing varicose vein surgery in a patient with sapheno-femoral incompetence and LSV varicosities

Position The patient is placed supine and the entire leg and groin is prepared and draped.

Incision A 4-cm incision is made in the groin crease just medial to the femoral pulse. The incision is deepened to expose the sapheno-femoral junction as the saphenous vein pierces the cribriform fascia.

Procedure This can be divided into three stages:

1 Groin dissection to identify and ligate all the tributary veins of the great saphenous vein before disconnecting the saphenous from the femoral vein.
2 Stripping of the saphenous vein by passing a stripper within the lumen of the vein down towards the ankle. The distal end is identified by palpation and an incision is made to retrieve it. The proximal end of the stripper is secured to the proximal end of the vein and the vein is stripped from the groin to the ankle by applying gentle traction on the distal end of the stripper.
3 Stab avulsions of the varicosities marked pre-operatively. This is done by making a stab incision and using a haemostat to dissect the underlying vein and gently withdrawing it.

Closure Haemostasis is ensured. The groin is closed in layers. The stab incisions may be left open. The entire leg is bandaged with a wool and crepe pressure dressing.

159

6 What are the complications specific to varicose vein surgery?

- Bleeding is very common but usually self-limiting. Patients should be warned of significant bruising that may last up to 3–4 weeks post-operatively.
- Wound infections.
- Damage to saphenous nerve with sensory impairment of the skin supplied by it, distal to the injury. Sural nerve may be damaged in surgery for short saphenous vein varicosities.
- Fibrosis of the operative scars that can produce hardness in the line of the removed veins.
- Recurrence.

7 What are thread veins and how are they managed?

Thread veins are thin cutaneous veins that commonly coexist with large varicose veins. They are usually asymptomatic and reassurance may be all that is needed.

Treatment is undertaken only after coexisting varicose veins are managed and may be in the form of sclerotherapy or laser therapy.

Vasectomy

1 What points should be discussed with a patient requesting a vasectomy?

This procedure should be offered to men who have completed their family. The following points should be discussed with all patients but in particular with younger men or those with very young children.

- Procedure is essentially irreversible.
- There is a small risk in the region of 1:2500 of not achieving sterility.
- Other forms of contraception should be used post-operatively until two consecutive semen analysis specimens are negative. (At 2 and 3 months post op)

2 How do you perform a vasectomy?

Position The patient is placed supine on the operating table. The scrotal skin is shaved and then prepared and draped in the routine manner. A choice of general or local anaesthetic can be used.

Procedure The spermatic cord is palpated and identified through the scrotal skin. A transverse incision is made in the overlying skin and fascia (see Question 5, Chapter 22, Hydrocele repair). The vas is identified and ligated between clamps. Care is taken not to ligate the testicular artery. The vas is then divided and ligated in two points and a small central section is excised and sent for confirmatory histopathology. The fascia is then closed over one end leaving the other end overlying the fascia.

Closure Fascia is closed as above with absorbable sutures. Skin is then closed.

The procedure is repeated on the contralateral side.

3 What are the complications specific to vasectomy?

- Infertility (if the patient changes his mind and desires to have children)
- Infection
- Scrotal pain
- Recanalisation of the vas and the subsequent failure of contraception
- Haematoma
- Testicular atrophy secondary to ligation of the testicular artery

4 What properties of sperm or semen are taken into account during semen analysis? What are the minimum acceptable levels?

Property	Minimum acceptable level
Semen volume	1.5 ml
Sperm concentration	20×10^6/ml
Total sperm count	50×10^6/ml
Sperm motility	At least half motile sperms
Sperm morphology	>30% normal forms
Grade of forward progression	Grade 2 (4 grades in total)

44

....

Zadik's procedure

1 Briefly discuss the aetiology of an ingrown toenail

The aetiology of an ingrown toenail is multifactorial. The condition is rare in people who do not wear shoes. Mechanical pressure from the shoe on the medial nail fold and pressure from the second toe on the lateral nail fold and onto improperly trimmed toenails will result in breaks in the skin of the nail folds. This is then complicated by bacterial and/or fungal infection, which results in inflammation and eventually abscess formation.

2 What conservative measures can be used in treating an ingrown toenail?

- Foot hygiene with regular daily soaks.
- Proper trimming of the toenails (square ends).
- Placing cotton wool under the corner of the nail to lift the nail from its embedded position.
- In cases of infection appropriate antibiotics can be given.

3 What is Zadik's procedure and how do you perform it?

This refers to a total removal of the nail plate (the nail) and the germinal matrix to prevent recurrence.

Position It is supine and it can be performed under a GA or a ring block. A rubber tourniquet is applied to the great toe.

Procedure Two oblique incisions are made from both corners of the proximal nail folds approximately 1 cm proximally and the eponychium is raised as a full-thickness flap. The nail plate is loosened and removed using a straight haemostat. The germinal matrix is then completely excised ensuring none is left behind.

Closure The eponychium flap is then closed and the big toe is dressed with non-adherent dressing. The tourniquet is released.